Confessions of a Carbohydrate Addict

Linda J. Gummow, Ph.D.
Robert E. Conger, Ph.D.

DEDICATION

To my fellow carbohydrate addicts. We are legion.

CONTENTS

ACKNOWLEDGMENTS

Without the inspiration and encouragement of my counselor, Barb Kershner, and the staff of Metabolic Research Center™, I wouldn't have recognized that I am a carbohydrate addict, and my excess pounds would still be with me. Without the comments and stories of other carbohydrate addicts, I wouldn't have understood how universal carbohydrate addiction is. I also appreciated the nursing staff, and I want to single out Cathy Windham whose gentle encouragement is greatly valued. I can't leave out my hubby whose support and writing efforts made this book a reality. Our fabulous cover was created by Robin Ludwig Design, Inc. www.gobookcoverdesign.com
Many of the photographs were from Pexels and Pixabay. We appreciate the creativity and generosity of the artists.
Thanks to Hunter Nelson who created our website.
Hunter.nelson@tortoiseandharesoftware.com
Visit our website. http://www.carbohydrateconfessions.com

CHAPTER 1

We're all on the belly boat together. — Unknown

What This Book Is About

If you're reading this, you have a 20-30% chance of being a carbohydrate addict like me. (Me = L. J.). Read the first sentence again. These words are telling. If you walk into any room with 100 people, 20 to 30 of them will likely be carbohydrate addicts. Scary isn't it? Thus, chances are very good that you're a carbohydrate addict.

If you're like me, you're also experiencing a terrible mix of negative feelings and self-references because you can't lose weight. It seems like others can lose weight. Late at night you ask yourself, "Why can't I do such a simple little thing?"

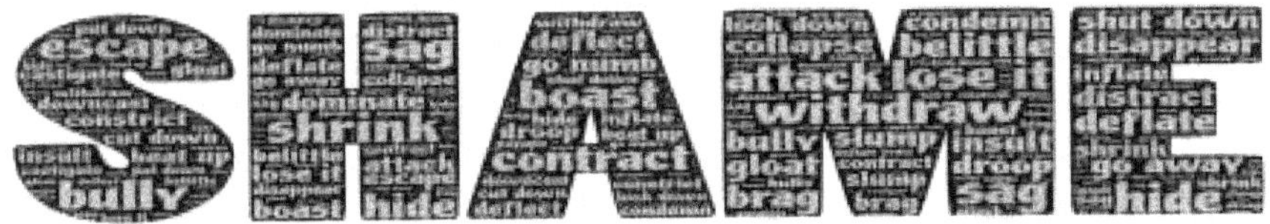

Image by <a href="https://pixabay.com/users/johnhain-352999

I grasped the magnitude of the carbohydrate addiction problem in the United States after I'd enrolled in a low carbohydrate weight loss program. I enrolled in a program because I couldn't lose weight no matter how hard I tried. Two things surprised me. First, I quickly lost weight without major discomfort when I reduced the percentage of carbohydrates in my diet. Second, my intense emotional reactions during the diet process were puzzling. My emotions rocketed from elation to anger. I started looking for answers. Why did the low carbohydrate diet generate such strong feelings? What did these feelings mean? Could anyone explain them?

I found a scattered body of literature related to the psychology of weight loss. Much of this hadn't been organized or reported before. Fueled by my anger, I started writing. R. E., my husband, supported my weight loss efforts, and he joined in the writing process when I realized that my curiosity had turned into a major writing and research enterprise. When you see the pronoun "I", it is L. J. speaking. "We" stands for both of us.

As I went through the weight loss process, new ideas cropped up each week. I often thought, I wish I had known this 10 years ago. What I was writing changed from angry rants to a desire to understand the lesser-known topics, things outside my awareness. I thought maybe others would like to know these things too.

The book is intended for carbohydrate addicts trying to lose weight and maintain their weight loss. Many of the chapters start with a rant which was triggered by anger generated by my weight loss experience. I felt betrayed and abused by a list of agencies and professions too long to mention. After each rant, I discuss related material.

Exercises are suggested at the end of each chapter. Your participation is strongly recommended. Passively reading books on weight control is like trying to learn to cook by reading a cookbook without getting into the kitchen. As the old blues song says, "You gotta get out to that kitchen and rattle those pots and pans."

WHAT WE DON'T COVER

- The literature on carbohydrate addiction is extensive and the research is exploding. There are better sources on the genetics of eating and addiction, neurobiology of addiction, food politics, sugar metabolism, etc.

• We won't tell you how much to eat on a given day. You're smart enough to figure that out.

• We won't give you any recipes to fill up our book. There are tons and tons of recipes on the Internet

PLEASE JOIN IN

Tell us your stories. Let's talk about our addictions. Others will benefit by getting to know your story, and you'll benefit by telling it.

http://www.carbohydrateconfessions.com

CHAPTER 2

My doctor told me to stop having intimate dinners for four unless there are three other people. —Orson Welles

I Just Can't Lose this Weight. I Don't Trust Commercial Weight Loss Programs. I Hate Me.

My name is Linda. I am a carbohydrate addict. Let's start with that.

Due to an illness and a prescription of prednisone, I gained more than 30 pounds. I had been slender, or nearly so, most of my life. When I gained a few pounds, I was usually able to get them off by cutting down portion size and eliminating snacking. However, this time, my usual approach didn't work. I decided that I needed to be more systematic, so I purchased an enormous calorie counting compendium. I went online, entered my personal data and got a calorie-count target for my age, height, etc. I then began counting calories. I did this studiously (and I might mention laboriously) for several months. I lost about nine pounds, but the process was miserable. I was hungry all the time, and I craved chocolate—my drug of choice. Eventually, I gave up. Of course, I then regained all the weight I'd lost. I tried this ridiculous routine several times until the fateful day.

My husband and I were doing errands. I was depressed and cranky. I looked down at my seatbelt, and I saw my disgusting belly (I named her Caroline). How she bulged over my seatbelt. I just wanted to scream at her. "Go away, I hate you." Then I thought, perhaps I should just accept her and go on with my life. Then anger, deep inside, boiled up. "No, stupid. Get help!" As fate would have it, we were passing by the Metabolic Research Center™. I knew nothing about the program, so I stopped and talked to a counselor. She explained the low carbohydrate/moderate fat-protein diet plan.

In the following days, something my counselor, Barb Kershner, said kept coming back to me, "I've read every diet book written, I've tried every diet, and this is the only one that worked for me." I decided to redirect the energy from my frustration and anger and put myself in her hands. Boy, I'm glad I did. I'm not affiliated with or compensated by Metabolic Research Center™. I am a grateful client.

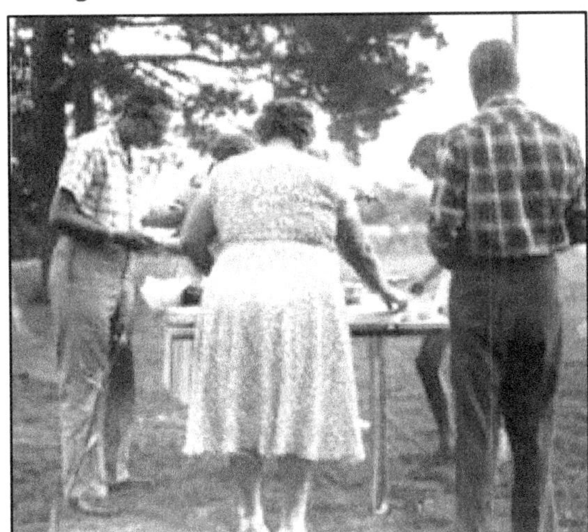

This is my now-deceased Aunt Caroline leaning over the picnic table doing the only thing I ever saw her do—eat. Aunt Caroline was a thoroughly unpleasant woman who delighted in telling me I wasn't pretty and would never find a husband. I decided to name my ever-growing belly after her. I decided my belly was not me, but Caroline. You can see from the photo that I come by my carbohydrate addiction honestly.

Rightly you ask, "Aren't there enough books on carbohydrate addiction, enough diet programs, and enough informational websites?" Yes, there is an overwhelming amount of information. However, most publications don't talk about the emotional experiences associated with losing weight.

I wrote this book on carbohydrate addiction for two reasons, one intensely personal and the other professional. On the personal side, I am writing this because I must. Caroline ordered me to. I awakened during the night feeling extremely angry. No past diet made me feel so angry. By training, I am a clinical psychologist. I had to discharge this anger. Plus, my emotional reaction made me curious. I wanted to learn more.

Obviously, I had to overcome my distrust of proprietary commercial weight loss programs if I were to have any success with Metabolic Research Center™. You know those programs featuring beautifully dressed actresses and other celebrities giving glowing endorsements of how much weight they've lost. These celebrities are paid, and they receive free food. They are really motivated to lose weight. Do they really eat the same food that you and I do? Even more upsetting are the back stories behind these celebrities and their diets. The most striking example is the saga of Kirste Alley and Jenny Craig. Ms. Alley became the spokeswoman for Jenny Craig in 2004. She weighed 200+ pounds when she started eating their products, and she weighed 145 pounds when she appeared on television. In 2008, her contract was not renewed because she had gained back approximately 75 pounds.

Given the glowing claims of the spokespersons of Jenny Craig, Nutrisystem, and Weight Watchers and the length of time these companies have been in business, one would expect that they would have data to back up their claims. Wrong! Do a Google search for long-term weight loss statistics and Nutrisystem's products. What will you find? A series of beautifully laid out pages describing the wonders of their program. No long-term studies. No studies by independent researchers. No statistics—nothing!

How successful are these diet programs in maintaining weight loss over the long term? I had to search the PubMed database. Tsai and colleagues did a comprehensive and systematic review of commercial and proprietary weight loss programs (Tsai, Wadden, Womble, & Byrne, 2005). They reported that Weight Watchers was the only program that demonstrated a "modest" weight loss based only on three short-term studies (i.e., three to four months). Since Weight Watchers has been around since the 1970s, this is no oversight. It is intentional. As for the other commercial programs, there was no data on long-term effectiveness.

After a 10-year interval, Gudzone et al. reviewed the literature again (Gudzune et al., 2015). They identified 141 commercial and proprietary programs. The commercial and proprietary programs with the largest market share included Jenny Craig, Nutrisystem and Weight Watchers. These three programs are high intensity and two of them rely on calorie-controlled meal replacements. Of these programs, Weight Watchers is the least expensive. There are several weight loss programs on the Internet (Biggest Loser Club, eDiet, Lose It!, Noom). Only 11 of the identified 141 programs had enough information on their effectiveness to be included in the data analysis.

Six of the 11 studies with adequate designs compared the Weight Watchers program to education only. People in the Weight Watchers program lost 2.6% more weight and maintained the loss over one year when compared to people in the education only group. Two studies compared Weight Watchers to going to a psychologist or psychiatrist for counseling. Seeing a counselor was as helpful as the best of the commercial programs. Nutrisystem does demonstrate some short-term weight loss, but no long-term data could be found.

Gudzone et al. (2015) discussed several self-directed programs which offer support through the internet (Atkins, Zone, Ornish, Learn). Of these programs, individuals on the Atkins—the lowest carbohydrate intake program—showed greater short-term weight loss and more favorable outcomes than the other three programs. However, clients who select education and counseling do nearly as well as Atkins clients (Gardner et al., 2007). The Atkins program used registered dietitians to deliver the counseling and education. SlimFast and Lose It! did help patients lose weight, but counseling is equally beneficial. Gudzone et al. (2015) commented on the weight loss achieved based on the dietary composition of the program. Low carbohydrate and low-fat diets were linked to the greatest weight loss at six and 12 months. Very low-calorie dietary approaches achieve short-term losses, but there are health risks and no evidence of long-term weight loss.

The message is even more grim when the long-term success of weight loss programs is assessed. More than 80% of dieters who try one or more diets regained the weight they had lost. Commercial programs like Weight Watchers, Nutrisystem, or Jenny Craig flourish because of successful short-term assaults on consumer's waistlines; however, these programs seldom succeed in the maintenance of desired weight loss. This leads many people to engage in multiple attempts with the same program before giving up. Some people return to programs 20 to 30 times, never accepting that the program has led them to multiple failures. The average weight loss for people who joined Weight Watchers is about five pounds. www.revolutionhealth.com.HTML). This weight loss estimate is based on a study tracking all Weight Watchers dieters—both those which stuck with the program and those which dropped out. Weight Watcher self-reported statistics only look at the average weight loss of people who stick with the program. Using this select group of patients misleads consumers. A loss of five pounds over two years is certainly better than a weight gain, but many of us need to lose more than this if we are going to maintain good health.

What are the takeaway messages? First, an angel was sitting on my shoulder on the day I decided to overcome my distaste for commercial programs and enroll in a low carbohydrate weight loss program. Even more miraculous was a fact I discovered during my weight loss journey. I had stumbled into one of the best types of weight loss programs available. Maybe it is better to be lucky than good.

Second, whatever television ads or weight loss brochures may tell you, losing weight is hard. Tomlimson described weight loss this way (Tomlimson, 2019).

Losing weight is a f---king rock fight. The enemies come from all sides: the deluge of marketing telling us to eat worse and eat more. That culture that has turned food into one of the last acceptable vices. Our families and friends, who want us to share in their pleasure. Our own body chemistry, dragging us back to the table out of fear that we'll starve.

Exercises

1. Name your least favorite body part. For example, I named my belly "Caroline." Wanda Sykes named hers "Esther."
2. Watch the movie *Eating.* It may be rented from Amazon. Was anything familiar?

CHAPTER 3

God give us glasses that make carbohydrates invisible —
Unknown

Please Tell Me I'm Not A Carb Addict!

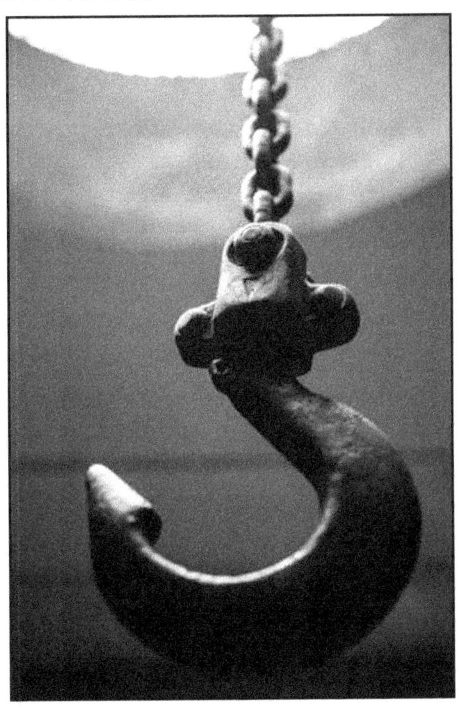

When I started the weight loss program, I didn't think of myself as an addict. I just had a few bad eating habits. Addictions were for everybody else. I wasn't hooked on carbs. I was just fine, thank you. Photo by Jaime Fernández from Pexels.

Approximately 10 days into the low carb diet, I was faced with a cold reality. It started with a dream. I was in a large ballroom seated at a banquet table covered with every imaginable size and shape of cake—chocolate cakes, German chocolate cakes, lemon cakes, marble cakes, apple cakes, carrot cakes dripping with glaze, and cheesecakes. There were several people, all strangers to me, seated at the table. We didn't waste time with introductions or interrupt our focus on the cakes in front of us with idle conversation. We simply dived in, elbows extended, and devoured the tempting delicacies. Gradually, we stopped using our forks and stuffed the cakes into our mouths with sticky fingers, ignoring the frosting covering our faces. Eventually, most of the cakes were gone, and the others stopped eating. A beautiful slice of lemon cake covered with white icing remained. Nervously, we looked at each other. Who would have the audacity or the courage to grab that last slice of cake? I balanced my desire to appear in control with my lust for the last piece of cake. After a lengthy struggle, I reluctantly pushed back my chair and left the banquet hall.

I awakened with a start. I was angry and confused. I had just experienced an intense nocturnal craving. There was no way to get around the dream. I was an addict. There would be other craving dreams and other cravings, but this was the champion!

✳✳✳✳

As I accepted my addiction to carbohydrates, I became even more determined to follow up on my diet program. When I repeated the dream to my counselor, Barb, she gave it a positive spin. I had left the last piece of cake. Maybe this dream was the beginning of a commitment to change.

Let's talk about my diet for a minute. The Metabolic Research Center™ diet program, their supplements, and their products are patented. See their website for details about their products. They have several programs, and the one I chose was a slow loss program high in meat protein. The plan is based on three identical meals. Each meal includes the following: 4 ounces protein, 4 to 8 ounces vegetables/salad, and one healthy fat. You eat no carbohydrates for 14 days. On day 15, you can eat one small serving of a carbohydrate or starch per day (equivalent to one piece of bread). The addition of a carbohydrate is closely monitored because some folks, like me, are more sensitive to carbohydrates than others.

I still hadn't fully accepted that I was an addict, so I decided to research food or carbohydrate addiction to see if there was some objective measure. I found the Yale Food Addiction Scale (YFAS) (Gearhardt, Corbin, & Brownell, 2009). You can download a copy of the instrument from the test developers' website. http://fastlab.psych.lsa.umich.edu/yale-food-addiction-scale/

The YFAS is being used in research studies around the globe. It is modeled on the addiction diagnoses of the Diagnostic and Statistical Manual of the American Psychiatric Association. The substance abuse diagnostic criteria are listed at the end of this chapter.

Individuals with substance addiction tend to consume more of the addictive substance than they planned, try to cut down or cut back on consumption without success, think a lot about procuring the substance, give up on important activities due to the addiction, have damaged emotional relationships due to the addiction, develop a tolerance to the abused substance, fail in role obligations like work or school, and experience withdrawal and cravings when the desired substance is not available. Intense feelings of failure and distress always accompany the diagnosis.

The YFAS presents 35 situations and asks the test taker to indicate how many times the situation occurred in the previous month. Based on the responses, you are classified as Food Addicted or not. The test results can also be used to classify the severity of the addiction (mild to severe).

You can take an abbreviated form of the YFAS online. https://www.cbsnews.com/news/are-you-a-food-addict-take-the-yale-food-addiction-scale-survey/

Yale Food Addiction Scale

Question	Answer	Score
How often do you find yourself consuming certain foods even though you were no longer hungry?	4x/week +	1
How often do you worry that you should cut down in eating certain ?	4x/week +	1
How often do you feel sluggish or fatigued from overeating?	2x/week +	1
How often do negative feelings about overeating interfere with important activities, such as work, recreation and spending time with family and friends?	4x/week +	0
How often do you experience physical withdrawal symptoms like agitation and anxiety when you cut back on eating certain foods?	4x/ week +	0
Do you sometimes keep consuming the same types or amounts of food despite significant eating–related emotional or physical problems?	Yes	0

Have you found that eating the same amount of food no longer reduces negative emotions or increases feelings of pleasure the way it used to?	Yes	1
Total		**4**
How often do you feel significant distress as a result of your eating or food-related behavior?	2 x/week	1
How often do issues related to food decrease your ability to function effectively, work responsibilities, social activities, etc.?	4x/month +	0
Score of 1 = FOOD ADDICT		**1**

Please note: I answered these questions as I felt before I started the diet program.

Let's look at my answers on the abbreviated version. Items marked "1" suggest a food addiction. Note: I answered "yes" to the item if I had experienced the event the number of times suggested each week or more. For example, I endorsed the first question because I was finding myself eating certain foods when I wasn't hungry more than four times per week.

When you total my answers on the first section of the table, my score is 4. A score of 2 or more means that I might be a food addict. The final two questions look at the amount of distress my dysfunctional eating pattern causes. I feel significant distress because of the way I eat more than twice a week. My eating pattern does not impact my functioning in any significant way. My score of 1 on the final two questions confirms my diagnosis. I am a Food Addict.

Last and most important, my inability to control my eating behavior is distressing. My dysfunctional eating pattern makes me depressed. When I started my diet, I didn't like the way I looked in my clothes, so I wore baggy clothes to cover Caroline. Wearing gigantic tee-shirts didn't help one iota. I avoided looking in the mirror. I was embarrassed about my food cravings. I began to hide food, so my husband wouldn't know how much I was eating.

I used to eat when I wasn't hungry. In my family, we always ate by the clock. My mother served breakfast, lunch, and dinner at the same time each day. She also kept a good supply of snacks and carbonated beverages. I have continued this pattern. I don't listen to my stomach. I eat snacks and drink carbonated drinks throughout the day when I am totally not hungry or thirsty.

As I am munching my snacks or eating my dinner, I worry that I should be cutting down. I do this at least four times per week. I do often feel fatigued or sluggish after overeating at least two times per week or more. Fortunately, my negative feelings about overeating have not interfered with activities. I don't have physical withdrawal, anxiety, or agitation when I cut back on foods such as chocolate or sugar. I do continue eating the same amount of food even though I feel awful while doing so. Finally, I am often unaware of what I'm eating until it's gone. Even foods like ice cream taste flat after a few bites.

Since I've been on the low carbohydrate diet, I don't eat sugar or most carbohydrates, so my answers are a little different at this writing. I am less distressed. I feel good about my weight. I know that if I eat rich sugary carbohydrates, my old eating problems will return in the same way an alcoholic can take one drink and fall off the wagon.

Your Relationship with Food

As most folks know, Body Mass Index (BMI) is an inadequate, but generally employed, measure of body weight. The BMI calculation uses your weight and height. To calculate your BMI, you can go to this website: https://www.nhlbi.nih.gov/health/educational/losewt/BMI/bmicalc.html

You may be thinking this book doesn't apply to you because you are thin or have a normal BMI. If so, pause before moving on. Think about the women you know. Some are painfully thin and others are heavy. These women may be of different ages, occupations, and ethnicities. Below the skin they have something in common. They are sisters under the skin. You might guess this by looking at them, but they could share a dysfunctional and highly emotional relationship with food. One woman may restrict food intake too much and the other woman might restrict too little. Some women diagnosed with bulimia or anorexia are perilously thin, but many of them would be classified as Food Addicts. These women's dysfunctional relationships with food have taken them in different directions.

Many women with a normal BMI have a dysfunctional relationship with food. I am one of these. In fact, one of my doctors was surprised to learn I had enrolled in a diet program. He said, "Your BMI isn't that high." BMI has nothing to do, I repeat, nothing to do with carbohydrate or food addiction. Estimates suggest that approximately 25% of high BMI individuals have clinically significant symptoms of food addiction, while a surprising 11% of individuals with normal BMI have clinically significant symptoms of food addiction. A whopping 57% of individuals identified as binge eaters have significant symptoms of food addiction (Gordon et al., 2018). What are the women who are addicted to food but who restrict intake doing? They must have developed strategies to combat their dysfunctional relationship with food.

Where does this take us? First, it tells us that eating disorders are about relationships. Food addiction is about your personal relationship with food. The rules of your relationship to food are yours and yours alone. No one else's experience counts. It doesn't matter if your husband finds that jogging solves all his weight issues. It makes no difference if your Aunt Sophie has kept her weight down by restricting her diet to grapefruits and avocados.

It might be difficult for you to see how anyone could have an emotional and personal relationship with something inanimate, i.e., food. Let's take a step back and talk about relationships between people. We're all experts in human relationships. We know that getting emotionally involved with the wrong person can be catastrophic. We're all good at telling others how to get out of their relationships, but we struggle to manage our own.

For the sake of argument, let's look at some components of relationships. Relationships are all about the emotions between people who are thrown together by choice or circumstance. The emotions can be intense like love or hate, or mild like friendship. Relationships have rules which are developed across time. Relationships often have rituals associated with them. Relationships are about preferences, what we like and what we don't. Relationships are associated with expectations. Relationships have to do with control, who is in control and who is not.

Think of eating in the same way. In our society of superabundance, we don't eat because we are hungry. We eat because eating is pleasant. We love food, and we love to eat. Think about a four-year-old boy in front of an ice cream display. The boy is excited thinking of all the choices and the delight of the treat awaiting him. He dances with excitement and runs from one end of the counter to the other. First, the chocolate ice cream beckons to him, but he rejects this and runs to the strawberry container. Often it is impossible for him to make a choice until his parents intervene. Adults are no different. Stand back at a buffet. Notice the bright eyes, quick movements, and eager expressions of the assembled adults. Notice also that some people at the buffet are more intense than others. Some merely like food, but others LOVE food.

Relationships are about rules. A relationship cannot survive without rules. Throughout our lives, we develop rules about what, when, and how we eat. Rules for eating vary widely by culture, of course. I don't eat insects, and the idea of eating a bunny rabbit is nauseating. Within a culture, individual rules vary as well. I have different rules than my husband. He loves to mix his food groups together. I find this repulsive; I want my foods neatly separated on my plate. No mingling please. He sometimes likes to eat dessert first. An abomination in my view. My sister curls her lip as she says the words, "I don't drink milk." This is one of her food rules. My in-laws, both thin and very disinterested in food, have few food rules. They will eat anything set in front of them with equal lack of interest. They don't care if the restaurant is serving Chinese, Mexican, American, or Indian food. What they notice is the people around them. They talk to the waiter, the people next to us, and anyone who will converse.

Eating has to do with rituals. My husband tells the story of a woman who cooked a gigantic Thanksgiving dinner for herself, her boyfriend, and her children. She envisioned a beautiful family sit-down Thanksgiving dinner. What happened was sad and funny at the same time. The children snatched a few pieces of turkey and ran to the playground. The boyfriend said he wasn't hungry and left to go drinking with friends. That left the woman alone with her ritual. Her answer—eat the entire meal herself.

One example of a food ritual and its relationship with emotional eating was provided by Tomlinson (2019). He described the aftermath of his sister's death.

What happens when someone close to you dies? People bring food. It arrived at Brenda and Ed's house, and my moms, within minutes and in great quantities. No matter where you stood, you were no more than 10 feet from fried chicken. I crammed everything I could onto my double-thick paper plate. The sugar and grease pushed back the grief, just for a minute or two, long enough to breathe. This is a terrible catch 22. The thing that soothes the pain prolongs it. The thing that brings me back to life pushes me closer to the grave.

Our food preferences are taking shape even before we speak. They are so much a part of us that we don't notice them. A family of my acquaintance eats this way. They sit down, pass the bowls in silence, serve themselves quietly, and set about eating. They lean over their plates, chew rapidly, and don't look up until the food is gone. When their plates are clean, only then do they lean back in their chairs and notice others at the table. My mother, being a farmer's daughter, scolded me when I rushed through a meal telling me I was eating like a farmer at harvest time. My husband remembers his paternal step-grandmother who tortured him at every shared meal. She required that each bite be chewed 25 times (and she kept count). Meals with her were a misery.

Our relationship with food may be obvious to the observer, but we are often unaware of it. To change our relationship with food and our weight, we must become aware. Awareness is the second step toward positive change.

Exercises

1. After taking the abbreviated YFAS inventory make a list of your problem areas.
2. Go to a buffet. Watch the feeding rituals. How do you fit in?
3. What were the meal rituals in your family? Which eating rituals are you perpetuating?
4. Are you angry yet? If so, start ranting! It's good for you.

SUBSTANCE ABUSE DIAGNOSTIC CRITERIA

The Diagnostic and Statistical Manual proposes several substances of abuse including —

- Alcohol
- Cannabis or marijuana
- Hallucinogens such as LSD
- Inhalants such as solvents and glue
- Opioids such as heroin or morphine
- Sedatives, hypnotics or anxiolytics
- Stimulants such as amphetamines
- Tobacco

The diagnosis of a substance abuse disorder is based upon a pathological set of behaviors related to the use of that substance. The pathological behaviors are divided into four main types: Impaired control, social impairment, risky use, and pharmacological indicators such as tolerance and withdrawal.

CHAPTER 4

You can tell a lot about a fellow's character by his way of eating jellybeans. — Ronald Reagan

Will Any of this Science Help Me?

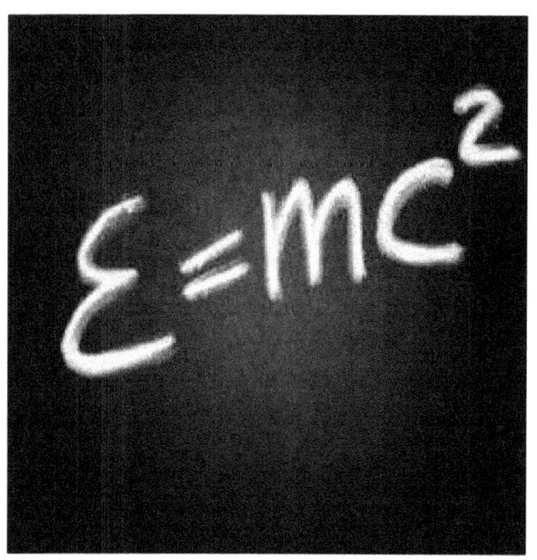

Every day I read some expert or another pontificating on weight and how to lose it. The next day, another expert says the first guy was all wet. Then, I find out that some scientists are "in bed" with food manufacturers and that their science was paid for by these companies. Scientists can't even agree on a name for my addiction. Scientists are debating the relative merits of these labels—Eating Addiction (Hebebrand et al., 2014); Food Addiction (Lennerz & Lennerz, 2018); Food or Eating Dependence (Markus, Rogers, Brouns, & Schepers, 2017); and Compulsive Overeating (Carlier, Marshe, Cmorejova, Davis, & Muller, 2015). The current term favored by scientists is Food Addiction. Carbohydrate addiction is a lay term favored by addicted individuals. Researchers use the term Food Addiction to be more inclusive. But we're really talking about being addicted to palatable foods containing Mr. Fat, Mr. Sugar, and Mr. Carbohydrate. I can't even conceive of an addiction centered around foods like broccoli or kale. Photo from https://www.pexels.com/photo/close-up-of-text-256369/

I'd lost confidence in science. This is how I thought when I started my weight loss program, but I was wrong. I am addicted to carbohydrates. I've learned that carbohydrates add pounds and pounds and pounds to my body while other foods don't make me fat. Although reading scientific studies is tricky, knowing some science will help you lose weight. How? Knowing how carbohydrate addiction works makes you better equipped to deal with your addiction.

✳✳✳✳

Carbohydrate Addiction Is Real

A lot of ink has been spilled arguing about whether carbohydrate addiction is real. We believe we've reached a tipping point on this issue. A tipping point is the critical point in a situation, process, or system beyond which a significant and often unstoppable effect or change takes place. An example of a tipping point is the rapid shift in public attitudes toward the heartwarming book *Divine Secrets of the Ya-Ya Sisterhood* by Rebecca Wells.

The paperback version came out in 1997 selling a respectable 18,000 copies. But then something dramatic happened as mother-daughter combinations by the thousands bought copies. By February 1998, 2.5 million copies had been sold, along with coast-to-coast national media attention. The tipping point was reached when it became a "book-club book" (Gladwell, 2000)..

Some scientists and practitioners will continue to debate the validity of the concept of addiction as applied to carbohydrates because that's part of what they do. However, the American Society of Addiction Medicine took an important step in legitimizing Food Addiction when they included Food Addiction in their list of possible new addictive disorders. http://www.asam.org/quality-practice/definition-addiction The American Medical Association finally got around to classifying obesity as a disease in 2003. This opened the doors for more treatment options for those of us who struggle with obesity. Many of the world's scientists are trying to find solutions to the all too obvious obesity epidemic. They, and most of the rest of us, have seen enough evidence in their lives and the lives of the people they love to have reached a conceptual tipping point. Carbohydrate addiction is real.

Let's begin, then, the task of building a model to better explain how addiction works and its relationship to obesity.

Carbohydrates Change How the Brain Works

Knowing how the brain is altered by the excess pounds we carry around will help us keep off the weight we lose. Believe me, losing those unwanted pounds is tough. But, keeping the weight off is the super hard part. I talked with a woman who'd been going to a weight loss program on and off for five years. She got the weight off, regained it, returned to the program, got the weight off, etc. Her explanation involved her family. They had different eating styles, and she eventually succumbed. The brain reflects what we eat, and it remembers our eating patterns even after we've reached our goal. To permanently lose weight, you must play the long game. How the brain works is a very important part of the carb addiction process.

The Brain Is Our CPU

Some of the early understanding of how the brain works came from cadaver dissection. In Mary Shelley's day, physicians were fond of dissection. Think Dr. Frankenstein. This fictional physician reflected the scientific thinking of the time. From the dissection work came a knowledge of how the brain is interconnected with the rest of the body. Eventually, scientists learned that the brain is the central processing unit for the body. For our purposes, the important part is that the brain communicates downward through nerve connections, and the body organs return information via several channels. These channels include neurons and hormones (e.g., estrogen, peptides, etc.). Scientists are still trying to understand and unravel the roles of the many interlinked channels of communication.

Brain and Body Interact with Feedback Loops

You need to have a basic understanding of feedback loops between the brain and body organs to understand the neurobiology of addiction. Let's take a familiar example, ovulation. This feedback loop involves the hypothalamus, pituitary gland, and the ovaries. The brain releases a gonadotrophic releasing factor that signals the ovaries to begin releasing estrogen. When the estrogen level in the blood is sufficient, the brain releases a different gonadotrophic releasing factor. The ovaries respond by producing progesterone and releasing an egg into the uterus. The uterus in turn begins to prepare for a fertilized egg. If a fertilized egg does not implant on the uterus, the uterus discharges its contents. The cycle begins again. If the egg is implanted, another even more complex series of interchanges begins.

Feedback loops are defined as either positive or negative. In a positive feedback loop, stimulation in the loop increases the activity. In the example of the ovaries, stimulation in the loop increases the secretion of estrogen. A negative feedback loop is the converse. A negative feedback loop would decrease estrogen output.

Different Parts of the Brain Do Different Things

The brain is a specialized organ. A lot of what we know about the parts of the brain came from the examination of human patients. These studies were often single case studies. For example, Phineas Gage. He is a famous patient who survived a puncture to his frontal lobes. Although he seemed all right at first, he was much changed after the accident. Eventually, we learned that the frontal lobes are important in the evaluation of information and in planning or executive skills. Another less famous patient had lost his ability to speak after an abscess was removed from his left temporal lobe. The infection had destroyed the Broca speech center of the man's brain. The control of speech is localized in the left temporal lobe.

Sometimes scientists were able to find a group of patients with a shared problem. The famous patient H. M. is such a case. Henry Molaison had intractable temporal lobe epilepsy. Henry's memory stopped when the tumor causing the seizures was removed by W.B. Scoville. For the rest of his life, Henry lived in a frozen moment in time. Even though he saw his doctors regularly, he could never learn their names. When asked for his home address, he recalled his pre-surgery not his current address. He couldn't lay down new memories. Studying people like Henry led us to the appreciation of a small structure underlying the temporal lobes, the hippocampus. Dr. Scoville's grandson has written Henry's fascinating backstory using his grandfather's records (Dittrich, 2016).

Due to the scarcity of human cases and the unpredictability of Mother Nature, scientists needed something they could control, so they turned to animal research. The scientist removed portions of the brain using suction or coagulation with electrical current. The animals were trained to do tasks that featured one behavior or another. The damaged animals were compared with control animals. For example, my second scholarly paper examined the effect of removing the hippocampus on maternal or mothering behavior of the rat. My poor rat mothers with bilateral hippocampal ablations were a disaster. They moved their babies here; they moved their babies there. Something important to maternal behavior was happening in the hippocampus. With the wisdom of hindsight, that something was memory mapping. Gradually, based on multitudes of studies like mine, a behavior map of the brain was being drawn.

How the Brain Controls Eating

So-called palatable foods (i.e., yummy foods) and drugs are both rewarding. These rewards are mediated by many of the same structures in the brain. From here on, when we talk about the rewards associated with eating, bear in mind that the rewarding effects of drugs such as alcohol are associated with the same brain areas.

Scientists knew that there must be brain centers that controlled eating and that eating must involve feedback loops between the brain and the many organs involved in digestion (mouth, stomach, intestines, pancreas, liver). Scientists started their search for a control center in deep brain structures close to the hypothalamus. This was a logical choice because the feedback loops between the hypothalamus, pituitary, and target organs were well known. Researchers began introducing electrodes into the brain's subcortical structures with wild abandon. First, there were electrolytic ablations. Then the concept of a permanent electrode implant was introduced. Scientists could insert an electrode into the brain of an animal, set up a behavioral paradigm, and observe the animal's response to the electrical stimulation. The current applied was low grade and did not damage the rat's brain. Rather, the stimulation presumably triggered neurotransmitter release in the stimulated area.

The breakthrough in our understanding of the reward centers linked to eating and substance abuse was an accident. Trying to study the reticular system, James Olds and Peter Milner inserted a thin wire electrode into a rat's brain (Olds & Milner, 1954). The electrode placement was way, way off, and the electrode ended up in the septum. Olds put the rat in a Skinner box, and he applied a small electrical current whenever the rat approached the corner of the box. He expected the rat would retreat from the corner. However, the rat kept returning to the corner. The rat appeared to be enjoying the current. They discovered that rats would perform behaviors, such as pressing a bar, to administer a brief burst of electrical stimulation to specific sites in their brains. The most sensitive reward areas were along the medial forebrain bundle. The medial forebrain bundle carries information between the ventral tegmental area (VTA) and the nucleus accumbens. Rats will press levers hundreds or thousands of times per hour to obtain brain stimulation in this area, stopping only when they are exhausted. In other brain areas, electrical stimulation was punishing and avoided. (See figure page 26).

Simultaneously, neurosurgeons were introducing electrodes into awake human epilepsy patients to map out sensitive brain areas prior to doing surgery. For example, if a patient had a seizure focus near the speech center of the brain, the neurosurgeon had to use great care when removing brain tissue in that area. Thus, the awake patient was able to report the sensations he or she experienced when specific brain areas were stimulated. When the current was applied in the reward area of human patients, they also reported pleasurable sensations. Rats, mice, and men have reward and pain centers in comparable areas of their brains.

Eating Is Conditioned by Our Experiences

Every student in an introductory psychology class reads about Pavlov and his dogs. In one of his now famous experiments, Pavlov rang a bell every time the dogs were fed. Eventually, the sound of the bell produced salivation. The dogs had learned that bells meant food. This simple demonstration illustrates the plasticity of the brain. The brain can be conditioned.

There are two types of classical conditioning that are important for the understanding of dysfunctional eating patterns. The first is classical taste aversion. I don't like to eat clams in seafood restaurants. Why? I once ate a bad clam. The taste was so unpleasant that I never returned to the restaurant, and I now approach all clams with caution. I can still summon up a vivid memory of the taste of the bad clam. In animal experiments, it has been shown that animals also learn to avoid foods that cause nausea, sickness or vomiting. Conditioned aversions often generalize. For example, an aversion to one shellfish can generalize to all shellfish. Aversive conditioning is particularly important in understanding anorexia.

On the other hand, positive relationships can be conditioned between foods and good feelings or events—positive conditioning. If a parent rewards the child with a hug and an ice cream cone, ice cream can be linked to love or good feelings. Take another more complex example. Your boss chews you out. You worry that he's going to fire you. When you get home, you eat a tub of gourmet ice cream. You feel better. Ice cream is now linked to both pleasure and the end of uncomfortable feelings. The very strong links which can be formed between emotions and foods help us understand dysfunctional overeating patterns (e.g., binge eating, bulimia, high BMI).

Can We Prove Carbs Are Addictive?

The answer is "yes". In an excellent recent review, Gordon et al. concluded that the "evidence supporting the validity of food addiction significantly outweighs evidence against it" (Gordon, Ariel-Donges, Bauman, & Merlo, 2018). There are significant neurobiological similarities between persons with food addiction symptoms and those with alcohol dependence. In an EEG study, participants with three or more food addiction symptoms exhibited brain changes like those of people with addictive disorders. Imperatori et al. compared resting state EEG brain activity among adults with obesity who endorsed more than three Yale Food Addiction Scale symptoms, lean individuals, and individuals with an alcohol use disorder (Imperatori et al., 2015). They found that food and alcohol cravings activated some of the same brain areas. Drinking a high calorie beverage increased activation in reward areas, the olfactory cortex, and the frontal cortex. The activation patterns were like those observed in persons with substance abuse diagnoses who were exposed to their drug of choice.

Why We Love Food

We love eating certain foods because we're wired to want them. Through evolution, brain centers developed to assess our body's nutritional status and what we were eating. Brain or reward centers were developed to tell us which foods are important or desirable. The brain releases feel good neurotransmitters (dopamine and serotonin) when we chew, taste, smell, and swallow food. Dopamine and serotonin are the heart and soul of the rewarding properties of food. Serotonin release is markedly increased when we eat the important energy food, carbohydrates. Dopamine, a neurotransmitter, is the chemical messenger involved in the reward center. Dopamine is released in the reward center when we consume sugar and other carbohydrates.

If you block dopamine as it's released, previously rewarding foods or drugs lose their power to reward or motivate. This principal has been demonstrated in several experiments. In general, the studies go like this. Rats learned to press a bar to receive electrical stimulation in the reward pathway. When the dopamine release was blocked with an agonist (or competitor), the rats stopped pressing the lever. In the absence of dopamine, the rats no longer found the stimulation rewarding. Visit the Neuroscientifically Challenged website and watch the 2-minute video on the dopamine pathways.
https://www.neuroscientificallychallenged.com/blog/2-minute-neuroscience-dopamine?rq=dopamine

A neurotransmitter is a chemical substance which serves as the principal chemical messenger between nerve cells or neurons. Neurons in reward centers in the brain communicate via electrical signals within the cell itself, but they rely upon the release of a transmitter to communicate with the neighboring cells. When a neuron in the reward control center is sufficiently stimulated, it generates an electrical signal. That signal travels to the end of the neuron, the neuron releases dopamine from its terminals into the gap between neighboring nerve cells (synapse), the chemical concentration of the transmitter increases in the synapse, and the neighboring neuron reacts to the dopamine increase by creating its own electrical signal, and so on.

Watch the 2-minute video to get a better understanding of the reward pathways on the Neuroscientifically Challenged website.
https://www.neuroscientificallychallenged.com/blog/2-minute-neuroscience-reward-system

Release of dopamine tells us rewarding food has been ingested. Most studies show that more dopamine is released when the food reward is sweet as opposed to protein. In other words, the foods we like (highly processed with tons of sugar) release more dopamine than less desirable foods (Berridge & Kringelbach, 2008).

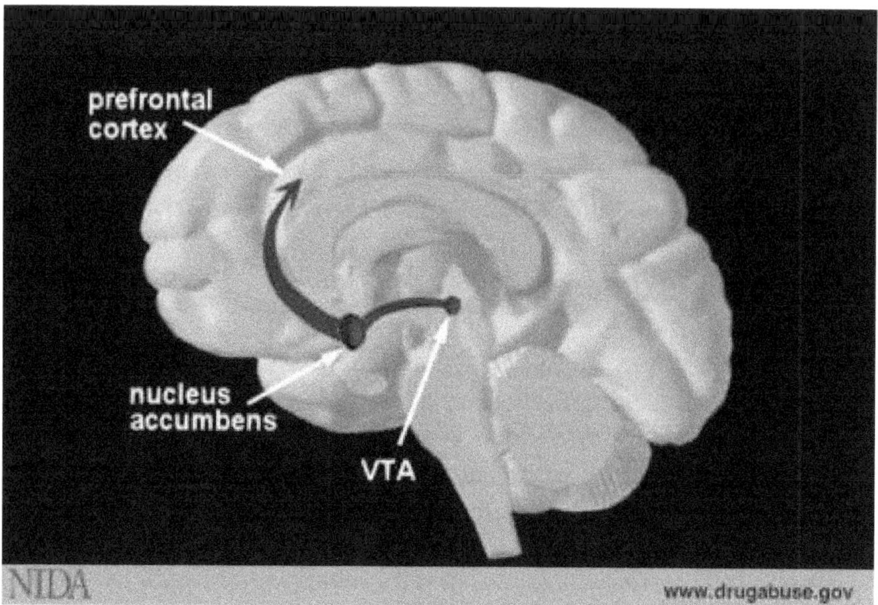

Activity in the mesolimbic pathway motivates us to seek more food. The mesolimbic pathway is important in reward-related motivation and learning (nucleus acumbens to prefrontal cortex). That is, activity in this pathway is involved in both getting you going to seek food, but it is also involved in establishing food preferences (such as my sister's distaste for milk). For our purposes, the conditioned learning of food preferences probably happens in the mesolimbic pathway. Cravings, such as my nocturnal cake dream, may originate in the mesolimbic pathway.

The second dopamine pathway is between the nucleus accumbens and so-called higher brain structures such as the frontal cortex and the olfactory system (involved in sense of smell). Activity in this pathway motivates us to plan to obtain food. The pathway from the nucleus acumbens is probably important in developing control over the eating impulses originating in the mesolimbic path.

We are over-simplifying here, but it might help you to think of the reward circuits this way. The mesolimbic pathway says "The body just buzzed me. I ate a wonderful bit of chocolate. Get more, please." The second pathway says, "Right on! Let's go to the grocery store."

Brain's Eye View of Food

As odd as it may seem, your body size makes a difference to your brain and how it responds to food (Lennerz et al., 2013; Gearhardt, 2011). For example, when a man with a high BMI looks at pictures of desirable foods, there is a strong activation in the nucleus accumbens. In the lean man, there is less activation. Gaining weight changes the sensitivity of the reward system. The brain of the lean man is not poised to act when pictures of food or soft drinks are shown. The brain of the high BMI man is energized, and he is more likely to seek a rewarding food.

Your pattern of overeating and associated high BMI changes the sensitivity of the D2 receptors (Volkow, Wang, Fowler, Tomasi, & Baler, 2012). Researchers compared the D2 activity of high BMI and lean participants. When exposed to a chocolate milkshake, for example, the high BMI participants' D2 receptors had a smaller reaction than did those of the lean participants. The sensitivity in the inhibitory functions of the reward center are reduced by habitually eating sweet foods. Think of this finding in this way. The brain's brakes controlling eating have been weakened, and the brain tells the body of the high BMI person to continue eating and eating and eating.

If we lose weight and want to reset our brains' view of food to a less destructive pattern, how do we do this? How do we tell the brain that we don't want to eat and eat and eat? Unfortunately, we can't answer this question. But our experience tells us two things.

Carbohydrate addiction is persistent and a bit sneaky. The addiction can pop up unexpectedly. It is as persistent as alcohol or drug addiction. Like the alcoholic, our addiction does not stop with a few months of sobriety or when we reach our desired weight. Carb addiction is always waiting in the wings, watching for a moment of weakness. When we lapse, the old brain circuits fire up again. In fact, carb addiction may be more persistent than drug addiction. One author suggested that sugar is more addictive than cocaine (Ahmed, Guillem, & Vandaele, 2013). Perhaps, evolutionary pressure explains why the effects of sugar on our reward systems are stronger and more long-lasting than drugs such as cocaine. Foods high in calories may have had greater adaptive value at a time when these foods weren't continuously available.

How we talk to ourselves about food can be the beginning of the end. When I talked myself into stopping for a treat, I talked myself into walking down the bakery aisle, I talked myself into taking just one, and my old habits carefully stored by my brain took it from there.

Exercise

As the folks in Alcoholics Anonymous would say, disclose your addiction to carbohydrates to someone important. Ask him or her for their support. My name is Linda. I am a carbohydrate addict. How about you?

CHAPTER 5

Sugar is for the body as narcissism is for the soul. Both pleasures kill. — Robin Sacredfire

How Carbs Make Us Fat

Why do they make it so hard to understand why sugar is bad for us? Who's the they? The "they" is all the experts we hope can tell us how to be healthy. They include the U.S. government's nutritional guidelines and pyramids (or plates), health organizations like the American Heart Association who are so deeply indebted to Big Ag that they have little credibility, medical researchers who take money from special interests and skew their findings, and so on. Photo by Kat Jayne from Pexels

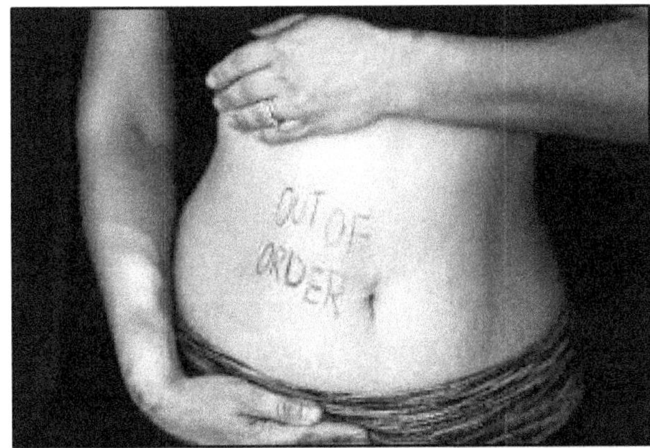

Why do they take something important and turn it into gobbledygook? The answer is money. The sugar industry is powerful because growing sugar cane is immensely profitable. The World Wildlife Fund estimates that each year 145 million tons of sugar are produced in 121 countries. Sugar growing destroys wildlife habitats, requires a great deal of water, uses large amounts of agricultural chemicals, and pollutes our waters when waste products are discharged. https://www.worldwildlife.org/industries/sugarcane

We live in Florida, and our unique resource, the Everglades, may never recover from decades of sugar cane farming. Tens of thousands of acres have been transformed from sub-tropical forest to lifeless marshland.

Maybe it will be easier for you to reduce your sugar intake if you think about all the baby birds you'll save when you don't add sugar to your coffee or buy that super-sized carbonated soft drink. This recent election cycle is the first in my memory in which politicians running for office are distancing themselves from Big Sugar and refusing their campaign donations. Who says we can't change?

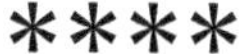

Sugar was once a luxury, reserved for special occasions and medicinal purposes. Dreadful concoctions designed to help the sick were sweetened so that the patient could get them down. That was then. This is now. We have gigantic refineries, and sugar is now so cheap that it's a throw away food.

Thinking about the history of the relationship between our government and Big Ag makes us livid. Two authors summarize this disgraceful history better than we can (Minger, 2007; Nestle, 2002). In 2015, after a 300-year history of working hand in glove with Big Sugar, the United States Department of Agriculture (USDA) finally recognized the health dangers of excess sugar consumption and posted the following recommendation: "We should limit our total daily consumption of added sugars to less than 10% of total calories per day." www.ChooseMyPlate.com

Whoa! Did we read that right? Usually, the USDA issues vague recommendations like "limit amounts" or "use sparingly". But the 2015 recommendation includes actual numbers for added sugars—less than 10% of total calories per day. This is still a bit vague, but let's clarify the USDA recommendation with an example. If you consume an average of 2,000 calories each day, only ten percent should come from added sugar. Your sugar allotment per day is a measly 200 calories. Sitting on my desk is a 16-ounce bottle of Coca Cola. Guess What? The nutritional label indicates that the bottle contains 220 calories of added sugar—my sugar allotment for the whole day. Help!

Sugar Consumption

There is obviously a huge disconnect happening here. Although estimates vary widely, Americans consume more like 40 teaspoons of sugar each day, which equals 640 calories (Zinczenko & Perrine, 2016). That's a lot of sugar! When expressed in teaspoons, the number seems nearly impossible. How do we eat 40 teaspoons of sugar? We'll answer that one by learning a few things about public health enemy number one, sugar, and the industries that deliver what we've come to view as a toxic material. Don't shrink in fear, Virginia. Yes, sugar in large quantities is toxic.

Let's look at the word "sugar". We think we know what the word means, but we don't. From the body's perspective, sugar has several meanings, and we lay folk as well as experts throw the word out loosely. We'll use the term sugar as a general class. We'll use the terms blood sugar or blood glucose when we refer to sugar in our bloodstream. The glucose in our blood is used to provide energy, measured in calories, to all the cells in our bodies. We'll refer to the sugar we, or manufacturers, use to sweeten foods or drinks as simply table sugar or sucrose. Remember, sucrose is not the same as glucose. The sugar in your bloodstream (glucose) comes from all the carbs you consume. This includes simple or refined carbohydrates such as bread, potatoes, rice, pasta, and table sugar. Sometimes media sources tell us we're consuming too much sugar. It often is unclear that the elevated blood sugar levels aren't caused by table sugar alone.

Our health problems come from too much sugar or glucose in our bloodstreams. Most authorities agree that white foods provide the largest contribution to the elevated blood glucose levels of many Americans—the consumption of refined carbohydrates including grains like wheat and rice, refined flour, and starchy vegetables. Refined grains are full of starch, a concentrated form of glucose. Each molecule of starch contains hundreds of glucose molecules. As soon as starch reaches your intestines, your digestive enzymes unhitch these molecules and release pure glucose.

Watch out for sneaky "health foods." Many commercially manufactured pseudo "health foods" aren't worth the energy it takes to chew them. For example, multigrain pretzels, power bars, protein shakes, etc. are filled with sugar and refined flour which release glucose into your bloodstream and wreak havoc with the insulin system and set off a host of metabolic problems. In other words, if you grind a grain to flour, it acts just like sugar. Avoid white flour, avoid white sugar!

When it's white, don't bite.

When Is Sugar Not Sugar?

Further challenging the carb addict are the numerous "hidden sugars." These are sugars that you don't see on the nutritional label but which the manufacturers slipped into many processed foods by simply calling them ingredients. See our list of some of the aliases manufacturers use to hide the amount of sugar in their products. Some of the aliases may sound familiar. But, have you ever heard of Florida crystals, diastic malt, nulomoline, drimol, or maltodextrin? We hadn't. Sounds like they should be in your medicine cabinet or your daughter's chemistry set, not your food.

Let's return to our bottle of Coca Cola to look at some of the hidden sugars each bottle contains. The ingredients in a 16-ounce bottle of Coke include water, high fructose corn syrup, caramel color, phosphoric acid, natural flavors, and 48 mg of caffeine. Two of the items, high fructose corn syrup and caramel color, are hidden sugars. We can't be sure about the natural flavors. Our best guess is that they're probably some form of sugar. These disguised sugars have all the negative qualities of table sugar and can lead to the same health consequences.

Don't underestimate food manufacturers, they are very crafty. This was a new one on us. Have you heard of "flavor boosters"? A flavor booster is a chemical which makes something sweet taste even sweeter. These boosters must act on the brain's reward system, but we don't know how. The boosters are listed as "artificial flavors" on labels, according to Senomyx, a California company that makes flavor boosters. Good lord, another alias to worry about! Sugar has more aliases than Al Capone.

Sugars of every kind and variety are sneaking into everything including health products. For example, Men's Vitafusion multiple vitamins contain glucose syrup, sugar, gelatin, citric acid, blueberry and carrot juice concentrate, fumaric acid, lactic acid, and natural flavors. That bizarre mixture went back on the shelf in record time!

We call label ingredients we've never heard of "mystery ingredients." We put a limit of three mystery ingredients per product. Watch out for artificial flavors. Who knows if these are some new form of sugar?

Sugar Meets Insulin

Not only are carbohydrates addictive; but, in excess, they make us sick and fat. A double whammy! In this section, we will outline briefly how carbs make us fat. The food we ingest is meticulously processed and regulated once it enters our bodies. Our bodies do the best they can with all the strange stuff we ask them to process. Our bodies can only do so much before they begin to show signs of strain.

Let's understand the metabolic process so that we can select foods which will enhance the success of any weight loss plan we put in place. Pretend we're eating a meal, say a meal composed of only carbohydrates and fats, a common occurrence. What happens? The digestive process begins by breaking down the foods: Chew, swallow, and send to the stomach to be metabolized. In the metabolic process, carbohydrates jump to the head of the line. They're digested and transferred to the bloodstream in the form of blood glucose where they are quickly used as fuel. Meanwhile, the fats we just ate have a different destination. They are shipped off to fat cells for storage.

Blood glucose derived from carbohydrates and sugars is the body's preferred fuel. If our diet is rich in carbohydrates, again common in the American diet, cells throughout the body burn the glucose as it becomes available. If we're eating more carbohydrates than the body needs, the level of sugar in our blood rises. Too much blood sugar in the system damages body tissues.

Insulin to the Rescue

To stem the tide of glucose, insulin, a dominant and multi-functional hormone, is produced by the pancreas and released into the bloodstream. In fact, your pancreas prepares to secrete insulin before you start eating. It's another of those conditioned responses we talked about, and it happens without any conscious thought. You take a bite, glucose begins flooding into the bloodstream, more insulin is secreted, and so on. As the blood glucose increases, the release of insulin ramps up as well.

When the body's energy needs are met, this fine-tuned feedback system uses insulin to remove the excess blood glucose. Any blood glucose not used as fuel will be removed by the insulin and stored as fat (joining the recently consumed fats) in fat cells. While this process is going on, insulin also "keeps a lid" on the excess store of fat. After a few hours, the body's blood sugar level drops and so does the insulin level. As energy and insulin levels drop, cravings for carbohydrates ramp up and the cycle repeats. We call this the "spike-dip" cycle. The dip in the cycle produces hunger pangs, cravings, fatigue, irritability, and depression.

Let's follow the spike-dip process over the course of an average day in the life of a carb addict. The addict starts with a breakfast dominated by carbohydrates such as cereal, bagels, toasted whatever, pancakes, or waffles. If the addict is in a rush, he or she gnaws on a fruit bar or a couple of doughnuts. The addict buzzes along enjoying his carb high for an hour or so until the mid-morning dip occurs. Now, he's famished and cranky. He grabs some O.J. or a power bar. He eats his usual lunch of a sandwich, potato chips, a piece of fruit, and a bottle of Coke. When mid-afternoon comes, he feels hungry and frazzled. Time to grab a candy bar and a latte. He sits down to dinner, the largest and best meal of the day. He eats a steak, a baked potato, and a salad or green beans. He's had a rough day, and the traffic was rotten on the way home. He eats a piece of pie topped with ice cream. About two hours later, he thinks a bag of chips would be a nice treat while he watches television. During the night, his stomach starts to growl. He tiptoes to the refrigerator and wolfs down another piece of pie.

During this 24-hour period in the life of our carb addict, the blood glucose spike-dip cycle was repeated several times. Count the number of cycles. The addict's body has gone through six cycles! The addict has eaten a diet made up of 60% carbohydrates—the average American diet. Each time the spike-dip cycle is repeated, the carbohydrate high reinforces our food-seeking behaviors, and our emotional state improves briefly. And, don't forget about the shot of serotonin.

For many carb addicts struggling with weight problems, the spike-dip pattern results in excess insulin remaining in the bloodstream over extended periods. If this spike-dip carb loaded eating pattern is continued, weight will be gradually added over time. Why did the addict gain weight? He gained weight by eating a carb rich diet that elicited excess insulin, and this diet prevented fats from being used as fuel. Rather, fat cells are added, and added, and added. I used to think that fat cells were like little balloons. When we eat too much fat, our fat cells grew bigger and bigger. Not true. Fat cells multiply. You get more of them. I find this to be a thoroughly disgusting fact.

As we continue day after day to consume refined carbohydrates and create elevated blood glucose levels, the pancreas tries to keep up by churning out more and more insulin to meet our demands. As often happens when things get out of whack, the body becomes less and less responsive to the glucose-insulin correction process. Insulin stops doing its job of clearing out excess blood glucose. This condition is referred to as insulin resistance. Insulin resistance is a precursor to a host of illnesses called metabolic syndrome which, in turn, is associated with Type II Diabetes. Not a path to follow.

Let's recap. Basically, carbs are metabolized and transferred to the blood stream in the form of blood glucose to be used as energy. To regulate the blood glucose, insulin is secreted and removes any excess glucose. After a time, both glucose and insulin decline causing us to become hungry and grab more sugar before insulin has a chance to clear from the system. Individuals with chronic excess insulin in their systems gradually gain weight over time. Eventually, they develop insulin resistance, metabolic syndrome, and other serious illnesses.

What to Do

So, what do we do to stop this tragic series of events? Prevention is a vital step in short-circuiting this process. Limit your consumption. Cut back on carbohydrates, particularly refined sugars, processed grains, and starchy vegetables. Restricting carbohydrates keeps your blood sugar *and* insulin levels in the healthy range, allowing your fat cells to release some of the fat they've tucked away.

If you are taking insulin or other medication to control your blood sugar levels, use extra caution when changing your carbohydrate intake. The balance between insulin, blood glucose, and carbohydrate intake is delicate. If you change the amount of carbohydrates you eat without considering your insulin level, you could experience serious consequences or erroneously believe that the low carb diet is not working because you're not feeling well.

For best results, work with your doctor and a diet center with medical support to check your need for insulin on a regular basis as you carefully reduce your carbohydrate intake. This precaution will cost you a few doctor visits and a few blood draws. Don't be a Lone Ranger and ride off into the sunset alone.

Learn who the enemy is and where he is hiding. Familiarize yourself with the list of hidden sugars at the end of the chapter.

Another thing to remember is to give your metabolism a breather. Leave a space between meals. This allows time for the blood glucose and insulin to clear out of your system. During this insulin-free break, the body can switch to the alternate energy source—fat. This healthy process is called ketosis. But, *if there is excess insulin in the system,* ketosis does not occur. We'll talk more about ketosis in other chapters.

So, put away the calorie-counting books and exercise machines. If you must count something, count the number of sugary carbs in your diet in grams—a number you want to steadily reduce! We won't say "Just cut back on carbs, nothing to it." There are massive challenges accompanying any attempt to "just cut back" on carbs. For the addict, these complications include a parallel neurophysiological reaction involving the brain's addictive responses. The blood glucose spike-dip cycle just described includes moments of intense craving and emotional high's and low's that are challenging to manage.

Sugarland

Carbohydrates surround us every minute of every day, all day long. This is where the enemy lives. We can't escape to another planet. Neither the government nor the food industry has much interest in helping us curb carbohydrate consumption. Big Sugar certainly doesn't care. They're in the money. Why change what's working?

In his book, *Zero Sugar Diet* (Zinczenko, 2016), Dr. Zinczenko mentions reaching out to over 40 food corporations with a letter. In the letter, he asked why certain products contain so much sugar when less-sugary brands on the market make comparable profits? Of the companies that did respond, 17.5 % responded with, "We have a variety of choices available." So, it's really your fault for choosing sugar-laden items. Ten percent of the companies said simply that they "were just giving people what they wanted." Again, you're at fault. A paltry 7.5% of the corporations responded responsibly with, "We hear you and we're trying to do better." Thank heaven. However, the vast majority of companies (60%), did not respond to the letter. Dr. Zinczenko interpreted the lack of response to mean, "This sugar question is scary. We're going to ignore you and hope that it goes away."

Exercises

1. Don't let food manufacturers off the hook. Consider activism. Write a letter to some major food corporation and ask them, "What's the deal with all this sugar in our food? And, what do you plan to do about it?" You'll feel better.
2. Take the list of Hidden Sugars with you when you go shopping this week

HIDDEN SUGAR LIST

Here are 80 sugar aliases. We think of these sugar aliases as food criminals. You will see these culprits hidden as ingredients on the packages of the foods you purchase. There are probably more sugar aliases, but this list should give you an idea of how massive the carb additive problem is.

Agave nectar
Barley malt
Beet sugar
Blackstrap molasses
Brown rice sugar
Buttered sugar
Cane juice
Cane juice crystals
Cane sugar
Caramel
Carob syrup
Castor sugar
Clintose
Coconut palm sugar
Coconut sugar
Confectioners' sugar
Corn solids
Corn sweetener
Corn syrup
Crystalline fructose
Date sugar
Dehydrated crane juice
Demerara sugar
Dextran
Diatase
Diastatic malt
Dried oat syrup
Drimol
Drisweet
Edible lactose

Ethylmaltol
Evaporated cane sugar
Flomart
Florida Crystals
Fructose
Fruit juice concentrate
Galactose
Golden sugar
Golden syrup
Gomme
Granular sugar
Grape sugar
HCFS
Honey
Honibake
Icing sugar
Invert sugar
Isoglucose
Isomaltulose
Kona-ame
Lactose
Malt syrup
Maltodextrin
Maltose
Maple syrup
Mizuame
Molasses syrup
Muscorada sugar
Nulomoline
Oat sugar
Organic sugar
Palm sugar
Panela
Panocha
Refiners sugar
Rice bran sugar
Rice bran syrup

Sorghum
Sorghum syrup
Sucanat
Sucroret
Sucrose
Sugar beet sugar
Tapioca Syrup
Treacle
Trehalose
Trusweet
Turbinado sugar
Versatose
Yellow sugar

CHAPTER 6

In politics absurdity is not a handicap. — Napoleon Bonaparte

Decoding the Nutritional Label

I wish it weren't necessary to write a chapter on how to read a nutritional label. Looked at from an idealist's perspective, the nutritional label is supposed to be an easy and convenient tool for consumers to use when selecting foods.

That's the world of supposed. The real world is quite different. Label reading isn't easy or straight forward. Here we show our skeptic side. The FDA gives lip service to providing helpful information while continuously working to make deciphering these labels next to impossible.

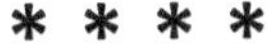

I've always ignored nutritional labels for several reasons. First, I don't understand them. Second, they're often written in tiny, tiny print and hidden in a crack in the packaging such that you must destroy the package to get a look at the information. I'm not alone. Most consumers don't study nutrition labels before buying food.

Due to consumer concerns about the steadily increasing amount of sugar in processed foods and the inscrutable labeling system, the FDA, at the urging of Michele Obama, formally approved a new nutrition labeling system for processed foods. This was the first change in nutrition label standards in 20 years. The old and new labels are shown side by side.

The primary changes are the following:

- Serving size is in larger type
- Serving sizes are updated
- Daily values are updated
- Nutrients required are changed
- Amounts of vitamins are declared
- New category for added sugars

Old Label   New Label

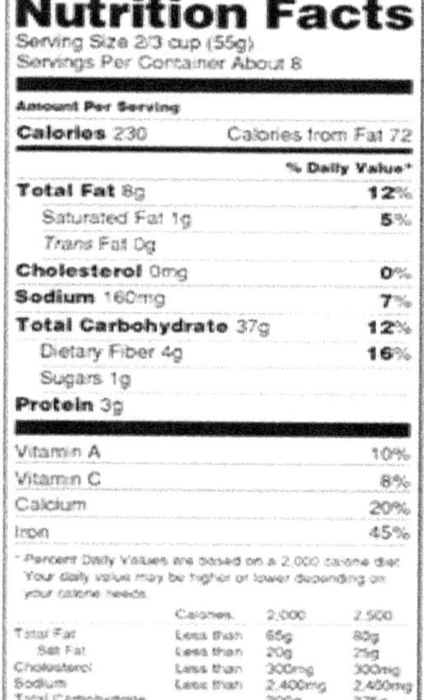

On the updated label, the serving size was revised to more closely represent the amount people typically eat. The daily recommended limits for sodium and the recommended daily values for dietary fiber and vitamin D were updated to be consistent with Institute of Medicine recommendations and the 2015–2020 Dietary Guidelines. Calories and serving size were made larger and easier to see. The amount and percentage values of vitamin D and potassium were added.

For the carb addict's purpose, it's the sugar category which is the most important. On the older label, sugar is listed in grams under the carbohydrate category. On the new label, manufacturers are asked to report two general categories of sugar—total and added. Natural sugars can be determined by subtracting added sugars from total sugars. Natural sugars are those found in unprocessed foods (e.g., fructose in fruits, lactose in milk, and so on). Because natural sugars come bound up with the nutrients and fiber of the food, they are generally approved in a healthy diet *within limits*. The example above shows total sugar of 12 grams and added sugar as 10 grams. This means that only two grams of sugar are natural, and the rest were added during the manufacturing process. Thus, natural sugars often represent a small percentage of the sugar in processed foods. Most of the sugar is added.

Another new label addition is important. This is the first time that manufacturers were asked to tell us the percentage of the recommended daily limit that this amount of sugar makes up. In the label above, one serving provides 20% of the recommended sugar we can eat on a given day.

How to Analyze a Nutritional Label

None of us have so much leisure time that we want to stand in the grocery aisle trying to figure out whether to buy a product or not. We use this process. Try it and see if it helps you make decisions.

1. Do a quick scan. This will often provide enough information to decide if a product is worth consideration. First, look at the serving size. In the example, the serving size is 2/3 cup or 55 grams. Second, look at dietary fiber. Dietary fiber in this product is 4 grams. Finally, compare the fiber and added sugar ratio. Here there are 4 grams of fiber for every 12 grams of added sugar.

   We follow Dr. Zinczenko's rule of thumb. In his excellent book, *Zero Sugar Diet,* he suggests that some sugar is okay if there is twice as much fiber (Zinczenko, 2016). This sample product does not pass Zinczenko's test.

2. Next consider total amount of sugar in a serving. In this case, there are 12 grams of sugar. This accounts for 20% of our sugar allotment for the day.

3. Third, consider added versus natural sugar. Here there are 10 grams of added sugar and 2 grams of natural sugar (Total = 12 grams). Since most of the sugar in this product was added by the manufacturer, the

food in the package bears little resemblance to anything found in nature.

4. Look at the amounts of fat (8 grams) plus protein (3 grams) relative to total carbohydrates (37 grams). This ratio comes out to be 11/37. Proteins and fats are significantly outnumbered by carbohydrates.

5. Look at the list of ingredients. Lots of secrets are hidden in this section. Check for hidden sugars, flavor boosters, etc. You won't find this information in the label, however. You'll have to look elsewhere on the package.

Based on our analysis, the sample item is not recommended for those of us who've decided to reduce our carb intake.

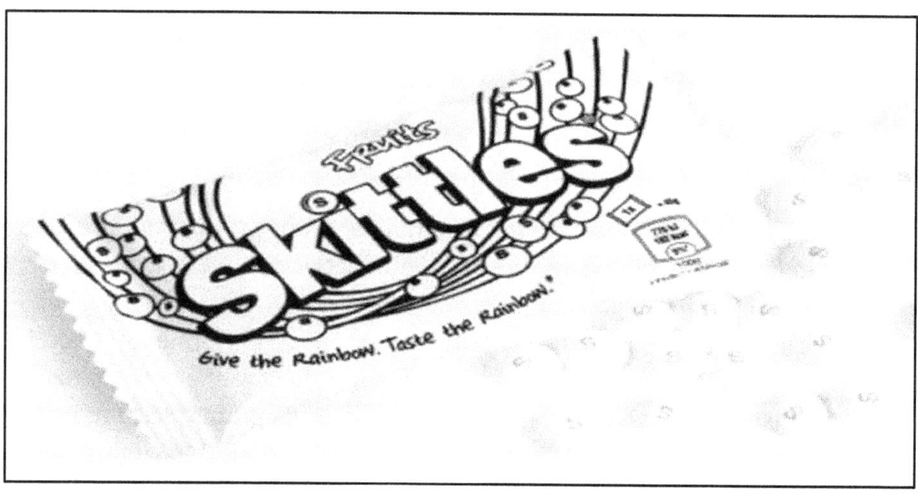

Let's try another example, Skittles. (If you're wondering about the black and white image, the packaging was changed by the company to honor the Gay Pride Movement.) We're not singling the product out. We're using it because I like Skittles. I used to eat them because I read the calorie number, and I talked myself into believing that there were 110 calories in the 3.5-ounce box. "Only 110 calories!" I chirped with glee. When I looked at the serving size, it was 27 pieces. When I counted the pieces of candy in the box, I discovered that there were nearly 100 pieces of candy. Ouch! Number of calories per box? 440 calories, not 110.

Let's run our analysis of Skittles.

1. Test 1: Added Sugar to fiber ratio. 21 grams added sugar and 0 grams fiber. Failed.
2. Test 2: If I eat the entire box, I'll have consumed 84 grams of sugar—more than four times the amount of sugar recommended in the guidelines. Failed.
3. Test 3: Sugar/Added Sugar ratio. Half of the sugar is added, and the rest is unknown. Failed.
4. Test 4: Fat and protein relative to carbohydrates. Skittles have no protein and one gram of fat. The ratio is 1/42. Skittles are not a friendly food if you want to reduce carbohydrates. Failed.
5. Test 5: List of ingredients. I had to get my magnifying glass out for this exercise. Skittles contain sugar, corn syrup, hydrogenated palm kernel oil, citric acid, tapioca dextrin, modified corn starch, natural and artificial flavors, colors, carnauba wax, and sodium citrate. Failed.

Skittles is an extreme example because it is a candy; however, this analysis can be applied to more complex foods.

One of the ingredients in Skittles deserves special mention—high-fructose corn syrup (HFCS). This nasty stuff is potent, extremely cheap to manufacture, and bad for us. More about HFCS later.

So Much for Good Intentions

When you look at nutritional labels in the supermarket, you'll find that some manufacturers have already complied with the new FDA guidelines, but others have not. The label changes were supposed to go into effect by January 2020, albeit, at the discretion of manufacturers. Manufacturers such as General Mills argued that these labels (particularly the added sugar part) were too hard for the cognitively challenged consumer to understand. Apparently, their concerns were heard by the FDA. The new labels may not appear on many products for some time, if ever. Since the announcement in 2016, the United States has a new president and new agency leadership. The first blow to nutritional labeling came on June 13, 2017 when the FDA announced that it would extend the 2020 deadline indefinitely. We don't know if this extension will be a roll-back or a repeal of the planned nutrition label improvements.

The roll-back happened without publicity. We, the consumer, haven't had a chance to weigh-in. If this roll-back of labeling regulations concerns you, write or call the FDA.

Reading Labels Is Hard Work

If you don't want to carry a calculator and magnifying glass with you and spend your life in supermarket aisles reading labels, you might consider the alternative. Shop the margins of the supermarket and buy as few processed foods as you can. When eating a packaged food becomes a necessity, try to limit the amount of added sugars to less than six grams. There are good foods mixed in with the poor-quality foods. They are, however, like hens' teeth—hard to find. The amount of time you spend reading labels will decrease as you identify products which pass the tests. Patience and persistence are recommended.

Exercises

1. Increase your awareness of nutritional labels when you shop. Stop and read before you buy.
2. Consider sending letters to manufacturers who don't use the newer labels. Perhaps if these companies knew we were reading their labels, they might improve their cooperation.

CHAPTER 7

I've been on a diet for two weeks and all I've lost is two weeks. —
Totie Fields

Faux Sugar: Use or Not to Use

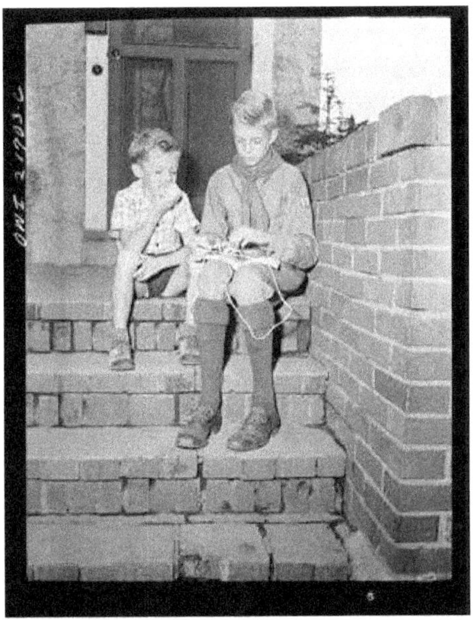

The literature on artificial sweeteners is complex, controversial, confusing, and chaotic. There's no motivation on the part of corporations, lobbyists, or governmental agencies to clarify and advise, leaving the consumer in the usual position of trying to make sense of a chaotic mess.

We'll start with sweetener names. Some call these artificial sweeteners or non-nutritive sweeteners. The FDA has renamed them high-intensity sweeteners. We use the term artificial sweeteners because that's what they are—artificial and created by chemists. To decide whether to use artificial sweeteners, we must unsnarl a dietary Gordian knot.

This picture, taken in 1943, shows a Boy Scout learning to tie knots while his brother watches. From the Library of Congress.

* * * *

Our apologies to Shakespeare, but the phrase, "to use or not to use," seemed to fit. Diet products of all types and description cater to our sugar addictions by substituting an artificial sweetener. We get the sweet taste, but we don't pay the glycemic index price. Is it safe to use artificial sweeteners? If you decide to use them, how much should you use? Which faux sweetener is the best? What about sweeteners that weren't created in laboratories such as the alternative plant-based sweetener Stevia?

The Rough Rider

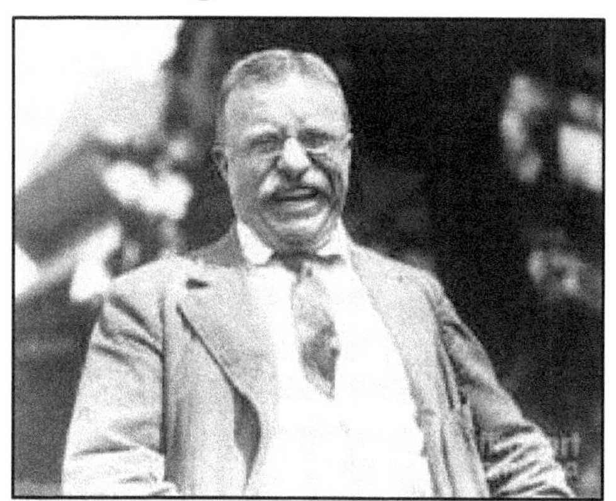

We'll briefly delve into the early history of the first artificial sweetener, saccharin. Saccharin, developed in 1879, is a derivative of coal tar. It's 500 times sweeter than sugar and can be produced at 1/10th the cost. Since saccharine passes through the body without being metabolized, it was recommended to overweight and diabetic patients by their family physicians. However, it was the "coal tar" part that put people off. Harvey Wiley, chief chemist at the USDA, considered the sweetener "extremely injurious to human health." However, President Teddy Roosevelt, fighting his personal Battle of the Bulge and a frequent saccharin user, retorted, "Anyone who says saccharin is injurious is an idiot."

The President had the last word. During the saccharine debate, Roosevelt put forth an insightful argument that remains cogent to the current day. For him, the use of saccharin as a replacement for sugar was the lesser of two evils. Roosevelt justified his position based on the trade-off: Sugar is unhealthy (as it leads to obesity); *maybe* saccharin is unhealthy, but we don't know. So, he went with what he thought was the less-risky option. We'll call this the Roosevelt dilemma.

The logic, then, behind the use of artificial sweeteners is simple. If you put saccharine in your coffee rather than sugar, you get the benefit of a sweet-tasting beverage with no added calories. This should, in turn, help you lose weight. Does the regular use of artificial sweeteners do what it promises? Do we lose weight?

Amazingly, after more than a century and endless debates, this simple question has no clear answer. By best estimates, 41% of adults and 25% of children consume artificially sweetened drinks at least once a day. Yet, after an extended search, we were unable to locate a single study supporting the contention that the regular use of artificial sweeteners reduced weight or prevented weight gain.

In a recent review article, Azad and colleagues performed an extended literature search. They conducted a meta-analysis on numerous studies related to artificial sweeteners and weight loss (Azad et al., 2017). A meta-analysis is a sophisticated statistical procedure in which high standards of scientific rigor are applied to numerous studies to separate signal from the noise (Silver, 2012). The researchers found 37 studies that met scientific muster. The best seven studies involved randomized trials, and the rest of the studies were observational studies, tracking the health habits of people over time. Most of the participants in the randomized trial studies were using artificial sweeteners and were enrolled in formal weight loss programs. Pulling these studies together, there was no evidence that using artificial sweeteners helped participants control their weight. In the observational studies, researchers found a small *increase* in BMI associated with the use of artificial sweeteners. There was also a higher chance of developing Type II Diabetes or cardiovascular problems. In short, there was no support for the basic argument that artificial sweeteners promote weight loss.

We scanned several history books to see if we could determine if Roosevelt ever lost any weight. Most pictures of him, as he grew older, suggested the reverse.

Safety Second

Since substituting artificial sweeteners for sugar doesn't seem to help us lose weight, is it safe to use them?

In the 1950s, the chemically derived product cyclamate was introduced by Abbott Labs. Cyclamate was considered an improvement relative to saccharin because it didn't taste as bitter or metallic. A combination of saccharin and cyclamate forms the basis for the popular brand Sweet 'N Low.

In the 60s, politics made things a little strange. In May 1965, the FDA and Drug Administration concluded that there was little to fear from cyclamate. Five months later, perhaps feeling the heat of competition, the Sugar Association published a one-page letter in the prestigious journal *Nature* asserting that cyclamate "could stunt the growth of rats" (at least if the rats consumed massive quantities). Cyclamates were immediately banned, leaving little question as to the political power of Big Sugar.

The sugar lobbyists' influence peddling, disguised as research, persisted into the 1970s. Using animal studies and massive amounts of saccharin, researchers claimed that consuming saccharin could lead to bladder cancer. This news produced a public outcry. Rather than ban saccharin, however, Congress opted for a warning label: *"Use of this product may be hazardous to your health. This product contains saccharin which has been determined to cause cancer in laboratory animals."* A second series of independent scientific studies failed to confirm that saccharin had any health risks, so the warning was removed by Congress in 2000. Saccharin was okay again, but cyclamate is still banned. Go figure!

By 2000, a multitude of competitors had taken over a greater share of the exploding market for artificial sweeteners, and new products were developed at an increasing rate. Aspartame is a good example of one of these new products. Studies investigating aspartame found no evidence of cancer-causing effects or damage to DNA. Aspartame was marketed as Equal. This was followed by the development of acesulfame potassium and sucralose which were marketed as Sweet One and Splenda, respectively. The Monsanto company (developers of the product NutraSweet) went to work on a concoction called neotame. Neotame delivered on two research goals. It was heat-stable, and it was intensely sweet (i.e., 7,000 to 13,000 times sweeter than sugar!)

At this point, we were totally confused. Who's keeping score? Who's approving and keeping track of these artificial products sprouting up like weeds in our food? We find them in one form or another on the table of every restaurant from Maine to Hawaii. The FDA, we were told, was keeping track. Great!

The FDA claims responsibility for the approval and safety of artificial sweeteners. To further confuse things, they renamed artificial sweeteners calling them high-intensity sweeteners. We would've loved to be a fly on the wall during that meeting. We'll bet the manufacturers didn't like the words artificial or non-nutritive tied to their products.

High-intensity sweeteners are regulated under the FDA category of food additives. The use of a food additive must undergo pre-market approval before it can be sold. The pre-approval process requires an opinion from experts who are "trained or experienced in the science of the field."

Currently, there are six approved high-intensity sweeteners in the food additive category: Aspartame (Equal, NutraSweet, 180 times sweeter than sugar), acesulfame (Sweet One, 200 times sweeter), advantame (20,000 times sweeter), saccharin (Sweet 'N Low, 400 times sweeter), sucralose (Splenda, 600 times sweeter), and neotame (7,000 times sweeter).

When the FDA classified the new artificial sweeteners as high-intensity sweeteners, they were way, way off the mark. They should have called these chemicals insanely intense sweeteners! These insanely intense sweeteners are food additives embedded in a multitude of commonly used products beyond diet sodas and breakfast cereals. These include, but are not limited to, coffee flavorings, energy drinks, protein shakes, flavored milk, fruit juices, flavored water, alcoholic beverages, dairy products, ice cream, jams and jellies, baked goods, gum, salad dressings, condiments, relishes, soups, candies, dessert toppings, canned fruit, energy bars, baked goods, microwave popcorn, vitamins, and probiotics. Again, this is only a partial list. For example, we found saccharin in our Colgate toothpaste and sucralose in our Crest mouthwash—both products were listed as inactive ingredients.

When it comes to sweeteners, sugar alcohols are the new kid on the block. Sugar alcohols, classified as nutritive sweeteners, are being mixed into processed foods. These sweeteners include sorbitol, xylitol, lactitol, mannitol, erythritol, trehalose, and maltitol.

Stevia and Monk Fruit

Besides high-intensity food additives, the FDA chart includes a separate category referred to as GRAS (generally recognized as safe). Currently, there are two sweetener products in this grouping—Stevia and monk fruit. They are both highly processed derivatives of plants, and these products are marketed under a variety of names. It's difficult to make any clear judgment about these products because GRAS substances don't require premarket approval. Rather, a GRAS determination is based on "scientific procedures that the experts qualified by scientific training and experience to evaluate its safety conclude, based on publicly available information, that the substance is safe under the conditions of its intended use." What this means is a manufacturer can make an independent GRAS determination for a substance without notifying the FDA. As the well-known author Gary Taubes put it, "The industry could freely use and sell them as food additives, but if new evidence came along to raise questions about their safety, the FDA would have to reassess them as well"

(Taubes, 2016). Obviously, the GRAS status is a kind of wait-and-see limbo. If a product has GRAS status, we consumers don't know if the product is safe. We only know that people haven't become ill or died yet.

The Mysterious ADI Chart

The FDA addressed the important question of how much high-intensity sweetener it's safe to consume by sending us to an Acceptable Daily Intake (ADI) chart. During the pre-market review, an ADI is established for each sweetener. An ADI is the amount of the substance considered safe to consume *each day over the course of a person's lifetime.*

In looking at the bizarre ADI chart, we did a double take! Who's driving this crazy bus? For example, the ADI for aspartame is 75 sweetener packets each day. It wasn't clear how this determination was made, but it certainly seemed excessive, bordering on the insane. Think of it this way, the ADI chart tells us it's safe to use a box of sweetener each day for the rest of our lives. That just doesn't make sense.

In her book, *Our Daily Poison*, Marie-Monique Robin reviewed declassified documents (I thought only the CIA classified its documents.). Her document review revealed "approximately 10,000 people spontaneously contacted the FDA to report symptoms they believed to be linked to aspartame" between 1980-1995. The complaints were wide-ranging—from chronic fatigue to seizures (Robin, 2014). This information prompted Dr. Hyman Roberts to publish a book which outlined the clinical history of 1,400 patients (Hyman, 2001). In addition to physical symptoms, over and over he observed an addiction phenomenon particularly in heavy users—complete with cravings during withdrawal. Dr. Roberts was asked if he had contacted the FDA. "Of course," he replied, "but the agency never got back to me. The industry considers all these cases 'anecdotal', even though hundreds of thousands are concerned" (Robin, p. 278).

We thought you might find the FDA's grudging acknowledgment of the possible adverse reactions to artificial sweeteners to be amusing. "In the event of an adverse reaction, stop consuming it and discuss your concerns with your healthcare provider." They provide a contact number (240)402-2405 for artificial sweetener users who experience adverse reactions. How reassuring! A phone number to dial on your way to the emergency room.

A culture of coziness is developing between governmental regulatory agencies and private companies. This cozy culture was highlighted by the recent crashes of the Boeing 737 Max 8 airplanes. A lengthy investigation by the Seattle Times revealed a close relationship between the Federal Aeronautical Agency and Boeing. In the past, safety inspections were done by the FAA. In recent years, the inspection is being outsourced (a term of art) to Boeing. Outsourcing is now a part of the regulation of food manufacturers. Food manufacturers are doing more of their own safety evaluations. In other words, the fox is in charge of the henhouse.

Why Artificial Sweeteners Cause Weight Gain

Scientific information is accumulating which demonstrates that substituting artificial sweeteners for sugar does the opposite of what we expected—they make us gain weight. How do we explain this paradox—we lower the number of calories and we gain more weight?

There are several explanations. These aren't mutually exclusive. The first common sense explanation of the paradox is "the license to eat." We think using artificial sweeteners gives us a little latitude. We saved a few calories on our sweetener, so we can eat more chips. We'll illustrate with an anecdote. A friend of ours, who worked as a checker at a local convenience store, told us about a heavy woman whose regular purchase was the following: Large bag of potato chips, five candy bars, a tub of ice cream, a couple of doughnuts, and a liter-size bottle of diet Pepsi. She confidently pointed out while putting the soda on the counter, "I'm on a diet."

A second common-sense explanation is how difficult it is to tell how many sweeteners are being consumed. Artificial sweeteners are often mixed with highly processed grains. These highly processed carbohydrates behave like sugar. They activate the glucose-insulin reaction process. Such products include all manner of baked goods from health bars to Twinkies.

Mixing artificial sweeteners with sugar-like products such as sugar alcohols increases our confusion. For example, the other day, R. E. picked up a little packet of a sweetener called Sequelle. Through force of habit (one he highly recommends), he immediately flipped the packet over to see the list of ingredients. The ingredients were listed as: "Dextrose with maltodextrin, aspartame." In real language, this can be translated as: "Sugar mixed with sugar mixed with artificial sugar." Separating out and choosing artificial sweeteners instead of sugars is impossible. It's best to avoid them completely.

The third commonsense explanation is that artificial sweeteners make natural, less intense, sweetness seem bland or even unpleasant. Remember the old song, "How you goin' keep 'em down on the farm after they've seen Paris?" Harvard Professor David Ludwig wrote the following:

"These synthetic chemicals stimulate taste receptors for sweets hundreds to thousands of times more powerfully than sugar, with possible detrimental effects on diet quality. People who regularly consume artificial sweeteners may find naturally sweet foods (like fruit) unappealing, and unsweet foods (like vegetables) intolerable. Artificial sweeteners may cause insulin secretion, driving calories into fats and stimulating hunger. Fat cells have been reported to contain sweet taste receptors like those of the tongue." (Ludwig, 2016).

I was bothered when I learned that overeating adds fat cells. Worse than that, I was appalled to discover that fat cells have their own taste receptors! I'd always thought of fat cells as rather passive. Now, I must deal with the fact that fat cells have wills of their own.

The explanation that artificial sweeteners turn on the brain's reward system has scientific support. When one of these insanely intense sweeteners hits our tongue receptors, they shout out, "Bingo! Yum, I've died and gone to heaven." The reward centers in our brain, now on high alert, scream, "More, more, more." The evidence for these assertions comes from functional magnetic resonance imaging studies and animal studies. When habitual diet-soda drinkers' reward center responses to saccharin were compared to those of non-drinkers, the reward centers of saccharin users were more activated or turned on (Green & Murphy, 2012). The effect of artificial sweetener intake on the brain's reward system is long lasting.

Animal model studies found that rats fed artificial sweeteners ate more and gained more weight. Their voracious appetites continued long after the sweetener containing foods had been removed from their diets (Swithers, Baker, & Davidson, 2009; Swithers & Davidson, 2008). The brains of the rats which had been fed artificial sweeteners were primed to gain weight, and the tendency to gain weight persisted.

The last and perhaps most likely explanation of why using artificial sweeteners makes us fat rather than thin has to do with how the brain and gut interact. The gut is an internal jungle filled with all kind and manner of critters. The gut microbiome is a vast and complex community of microbes lining our intestinal tract. Suez and colleagues have studied the interaction between the microbiome and sweeteners using animals. In a recent article in *Nature*, the authors wrote: "Here we demonstrate that consumption of commonly used NAS (artificial sweeteners) formulations drives the development of glucose intolerance induction of compositional and functional alterations of the intestinal microbiota" (Suez et al., 2014).

Let's decode that nearly unintelligible sentence. When nature is left to her own devices, the sweet taste of foods predicts its energy content. In general, the sweeter the taste, the higher the energy density. In other words, the gut is built to expect to receive energy in proportion to the sweetness of the foods we eat. When we use artificial sweeteners, this relationship no longer holds. The food tastes sweet, the tongue and brain interpret the food as sweet, but the food doesn't provide the anticipated energy to the gut and all the microbiota living in it. Let's look at fruit, for example. Fruits are viscous. The viscosity of the food usually parallels its sweetness. Over eons of evolution, organisms have learned to adjust their intake based upon the expected caloric content of foods.

Enter the era of sweetened and artificially sweetened beverages and foods. These foods and beverages are sweet, but they don't supply energy. Particularly dangerous are super sweetened beverages which further disturb our body's expectations. Our bodies cannot predict the caloric consequences of what we eat.

In rats, there is evidence that the weakening of the association between sweet taste and energy content increases body weight. The ability of rat pups to maintain a stable weight was disrupted by saccharin exposure. Altering the normal predictive relationship between sweet taste, food viscosity, and calories may contribute to overeating and weight gain. Those of us who use artificial sweeteners can't judge caloric or energy intake. The link between taste, reward, and carbohydrate metabolism is altered, and this leads to a profound change in how our bodies regulate energy. Also, by changing the links between sweet tasting carbohydrates and energy, we change the reward system of our brains. Davidson and Swithers (2004) suggest that loss of our ability to use the sweetness of foods to predict the caloric consequences of their intake contributes to overeating and excessive weight gain.

Consuming too many artificially sweetened foods and drinks makes us fat. Accept this, however hateful.

Diet Soda & Artificial Sweeteners: Does Amount Matter?

If you decide to use artificial sweeteners, does the amount of sweetener consumed matter? Although there is no definitive answer, what we do know is that one would be wise to use as little artificial sweetener as possible. There is some information on the relationship between the amount of diet soda consumed and the alterations in the brain's reward system. Activation in response to saccharin is highly associated with the number of diet sodas consumed per week. One diet soda a day may produce a small change, but four diet sodas each day makes a large change (Rudenga, 2012). "Taken together, these results suggest that regular consumption of diet soda may be related to alterations in the reward experienced by both nutritive and nonnutritive sweet taste." One diet soda per day probably won't do much harm, particularly if the soda is taken with food, but five diet sodas per day is four too many.

Can artificial sweeteners and added sweeteners hold our brains captive? The answer is "yes". Sadly, heavy use of super sweet artificial or super sweeteners is linked to carbohydrate addiction. In one study, the intense sweetness of artificial sweeteners surpassed the rewarding effects of cocaine in the brain (Lenoir & Fuschia, 2007). The "supranormal" stimulation provided by artificially sweetened foods generates supranormal reward signals in the brain. The supranormal reward signals can override our "self-control mechanisms" and lead to addiction.

How do we resolve the Roosevelt dilemma, saccharin vs. sugar? Perhaps by saying, "Hey, wait a minute. There's a third alternative. How about neither?" Of course, many people have made this choice, but the just-say-no group remains in the distinct minority. We hope you'll consider building a future without sugar substitutes or excessive sugar intake. Foods taste incredible when they're not overshadowed by pumped up Snickers bars.

Exercises

1. Sugars and artificial sweeteners are mixed into processed foods. In fact, it's nearly impossible to find packaged food without some type

of sweetener. Each time you walk through the supermarket, look at the nutritional label on a packaged food you commonly purchase. How many artificial sweeteners or sugars do you find?

2. Does the thought of giving up artificial sweeteners make you sweat? If so, consider tracking your artificial sweetener intake and gradually cutting back. As a reformed Coca Cola drinker, I can tell you that your sense of taste will adjust to less sweetness and will eventually find super sweet foods to be nauseating.

CHAPTER 8

*Mothers, food, love, and career, the four major guilt groups. —
Cathy Guisewite*

How Did Fat Get a Bad Rap?

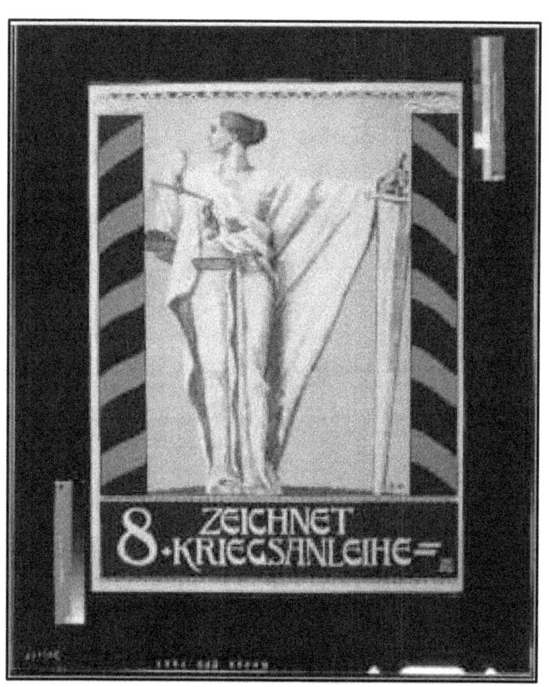

If I were to write everything I've heard about the horrors of fat consumption, I'd go on for pages. I'll tell you my story instead. My doctor told me I should watch my cholesterol. I cut eggs, dairy, cheese, etc. from my diet. I scrupulously removed the skin from my chicken and reduced my intake of beef. I stopped using butter and substituted olive oil or canola oil. I no longer ate avocados. I studied low fat cookbooks by the American Heart Association. As I munched away on all manner of carbohydrates, I felt very superior to the poor slobs who mindlessly slurped down their greasy steak and whole milk. Photo of Justice from a poster in the Library of Congress

Then I found out about the low carbohydrate diet, and it turned my world upside down. My counselor told me fat was good for me! Eating fat could even promote weight loss. As the pounds dropped off each week and I experienced no hunger pangs, a burning rage developed. I could talk of nothing else. How could I have been so wrong? How could my doctor, the American Heart Association, and nutritional experts have led me so far astray? Wasn't there anyone at the wheel when this travesty against our health was committed?

* * * *

Definitions

Let's look at how fat became a dietary bad boy. We've drawn heavily from the excellent works of Marion Nestle, Denise Minger, Nina Teicholz, and Gary Taubes (Minger, 2007; Nestle, 2002; Teicholz, 2014; Taubes, 2016; Taubes, 2001).

When we talk about fat, we aren't necessarily using the same meaning. To help you make sense of what follows, let's start with some definitions. The characters in the health drama—triglycerides, cholesterol, and lipoproteins—are shown in the table. The compound and its general functions are listed.

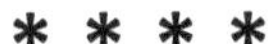

Types of Lipids or Fats

- Triglycerides
    Energy storage in fat cells, carried in blood by VLDL
- Cholesterol
    Builds cell membranes, steroid hormones
    carried in blood by LDL & HDL
- Lipoproteins
    Molecules of lipid assembled with protein
    Transport vehicles for triglycerides and cholesterol
        LDL-low density lipoprotein
        HDL-high density lipoprotein
        VLDL-very low density lipoprotein

Fat is a lipid. Fat cells release triglycerides into the blood stream when they are needed for energy. The triglycerides are transported to their destinations by very low-density lipoprotein or VLDL. Cholesterol is obtained from the foods we eat or is manufactured by the liver. Cholesterol has several functions including building cell membranes and serving as a base for steroid hormone manufacture. Cholesterol is carried in the blood by either low density lipoprotein (LDL) or high-density lipoprotein (HDL). Lipoproteins are a combination of lipids and protein. They are transport molecules. There are three categories based upon density—low density, high density, and very low density.

As we all know, fat is part of the foods we eat. These fats are defined and discussed later.

Fat's Sad Fall from Grace

The story of fat's fall from grace begins in the early 1950s. Although fat had been treated with downright suspicion for centuries, the vilification of fat began in earnest in the 1950s with the publication of the infamous *Six Countries Study* by Ansel Keys. Keys was a scientist, pioneer, promoter, policymaker, and author. But mostly, he was high strung, brash, opinionated, rigid, and biased. He believed that fat was a health villain. What drove his beliefs was the epidemic of heart attacks in the 1940s. These attacks, affecting primarily middle-aged men, were surprise attacks which included sudden tightening of the chest, collapsing into unconsciousness, and occasionally followed by coma and death. If the victim survived, he had a high risk of additional attacks. Several characteristics linked the heart attack victims. They were overweight, sedentary, and employed in high-pressure jobs.

Researchers later found that heart attack victims had another characteristic in common—cholesterol in atherosclerotic plaques in their blood vessels. Cholesterol had built up along the narrow artery walls until the blood supply to the heart was nearly shut off. The image of a yellow heap of fat piling up in the highways leading to your heart is compelling. There had to be a link between these attacks and the nasty yellow stuff in the arteries. Scientists discussed the possibility of preventing heart attacks by stopping the waxy build up.

The next step in Keys' logic was simple. How does cholesterol get into the body? It had to come from foods. Researchers looked at foods which might influence the amount of cholesterol in the bloodstream. They discovered that replacing animal fats with vegetable fats lowered total blood cholesterol. Animal fats, found in lard and dairy products such as butter, contain high levels of saturated fats. As these investigations continued, Keys began to consider all fats—including those found in plants—to be problematic.

However, he decided saturated fats were public health enemy number one. But where was his proof?

Six Countries Study

In 1952, Keys unveiled his *Six Countries Study.* Starting with the presumption of a strong relationship between dietary fat consumption and deaths from heart disease, Keys and his colleagues collected data from 22 countries to test this notion. If Keys and colleagues couldn't find the data they wanted, they used estimates. As well, they narrowed their selection to six countries in which the data supported their assumption. In other words, they fudged the data and then engaged in cherry-picking! Keys selected Italy, England, Australia, Canada, Japan, and the United States to test his assumption.

Keys declared that the varied dietary habits in the countries selected supported his diet-heart hypothesis. In countries like the United States and Great Britain, which Keys said consumed more fat, the incidence of heart disease was greater than in countries which ate less fat (e.g., Japan). In the figure, death by heart disease (incidence per 1,000) is designated by black bars. The checked bars show the percentage of the population's diet which was made up of fat. In Japan, both heart disease and fat consumption were negligible, but Canadian and US data suggested support for the diet-heart hypothesis.

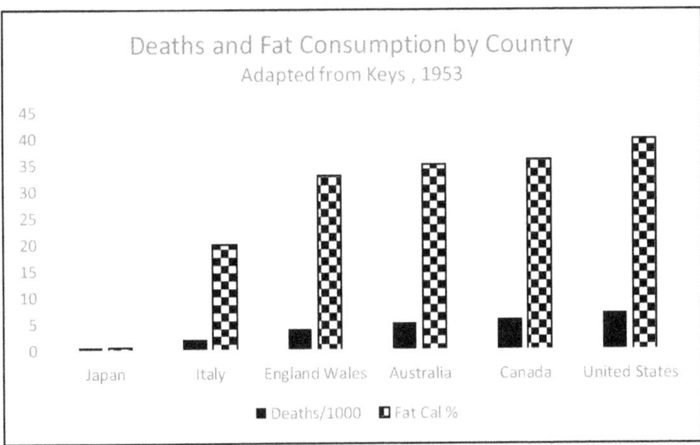

Beyond the flawed data and cherry-picking approach, there were other problems with the *Six Countries Study*, not least of which was the correlational nature of the data analysis. As even beginning researchers are aware, correlation does not mean causation. Despite considerable criticism from the scientific community about the *Six Countries Study*, Keys was on a mission and not to be denied.

Over the years, Keys' diet-heart hypothesis grew in popularity. Big Sugar loved the idea and so did the medical-pharmaceutical industrial complex. The race was on: Find a drug which would lower the dreaded blood cholesterol. The medication class, statins, lowered serum cholesterol. When blood cholesterol lowering drugs hit the market in the 1980s, there was a billion-dollar payoff to pharmaceutical companies. Also, food manufacturers capitalized on every variety of low-fat product from yogurt to energy bars by taking the fat out and adding sugar to improve taste. Physicians and health counselors recommended cutting back on animal meats, eggs, and dairy products. In their place, processed grains, bread, pasta, cereal, and skim milk were recommended.

Although large-scale studies were funded to confirm the diet-heart hypothesis, they generally produced mixed or negative results. Several studies were seriously flawed (Leren, 1970 Oslo Diet-Heart study; 1969 The Los Angeles Veteran's Administration study; Turpeinen, 1979 The Finnish Mental Hospital study; 1982 the Multiple Risk-Factor Intervention Trial; Prentice, 2017; The Women's Health Initiative, 1993). For supporters of the diet-heart disease hypothesis, the results of the Women's Health Initiative (WHI) 10-year follow-up study were disappointing. The WHI was the largest and longest study of the low-fat diet ever undertaken, the Rolls Royce of studies. In the WHI study, subjects in the low-fat diet group were just as likely to be diagnosed with heart disease, stroke, and cancer. In addition, subjects on the low-fat diet didn't lose weight. The low-fat diet hadn't made a dent in heart disease or any other ailment.

The flaws in the simplistic cholesterol hypothesis are clear when one looks at the routine health examinations undergone by millions of Americans each year. Rather than simply searching for Keys' public enemy number one, cholesterol, the examination currently includes a complex series of tests called a lipid panel. This panel considers the contributions of cholesterol, triglycerides, HDL (good cholesterol), LDL (bad cholesterol), and VLDL. Combinations of these various substances (e.g., VLDL and triglycerides) and ratios of substances (HDL-to-LDL) may be taken into consideration. In select cases, an evaluation of the density of LDL particles may be ordered.

Physicians are now aware that high levels of triglycerides in the blood can increase your heart disease risk. Like cholesterol, triglycerides are a type of fat found in your blood stream. While glucose is being used as fuel, triglycerides are stored in fat cells, with insulin keeping the lid on. Between meals, when insulin levels decline, triglycerides are released to be burned as fuel in a process called ketosis.

The lipoproteins, HDL (good) and LDL (bad) transport cholesterol throughout the body. HDL is referred to as good because one of its functions is to clear the buildup of fatty plaques in your arteries. After completing its transport task, LDL is removed from the bloodstream by scavenger cells called macrophages. The LDL particles and macrophages that engulf them tend to bind to the artery walls, elevating the risk for cardiovascular disease.

The lipoprotein VLDL enters the picture in combination with triglycerides. Researchers have determined that smaller LDL particles can slip through the tiny openings between the cells lining your arteries. This discovery has prompted another and more refined level of cardio-risk assessment. That is, a high concentration of small, dense LDL particles can be a predictor of cardiovascular disease, even when LDL readings are in the normal range.

In addition to the lipid panel, a skilled clinician must take a variety of family and demographic risk factors into consideration before advancing a diagnosis of cardiovascular disease. The process is not a simple task of assigning a cholesterol cut-off score and making a diagnosis based on a single number, as the diet heart disease hypothesis suggested.

Teicholz (2014) concluded, "The inescapable conclusion from numerous trials on this (low-fat) diet, altogether costing more than $1 billion, can only be that this regime, which became our national diet before being properly tested, has almost certainly been a terrible mistake for American public health."

Thus, as the 20th Century ended, scientific experts, government officials, food industry execs, Big Pharma, and medical associations clung to the low-fat paradigm while most of the population—men, women and children—continued to gain weight and worried about their increasingly fat bellies.

Enter the Mediterranean Diet

The Mediterranean Diet, featuring olive oil in a starring role, made a brief appearance in the 1990s, but it faded out due to lack of definition. In fact, promoters of the Mediterranean diet never really settled on a definition of what it was or was not. If you look at countries bordering the Mediterranean Sea, you'll notice a rather complicated grouping: Egypt, Israel, Lebanon, Syria, Turkey, Greece, Albania, Italy, France, Andorra, Spain, Morocco, Algeria, Libya, and tiny Morocco. Getting this group together to agree on much of anything, including diet, would seem a risky endeavor.

An important evaluation of the Mediterranean diet, however, was conducted in Israel in 2008. This well-designed and rigorous random-trial study was conducted by an international group of researchers (Shai et al., 2008). The researchers selected 322 moderately obese middle-aged subjects and put them on one of three diets: The traditional low-fat diet, the Mediterranean diet, and a low-carbohydrate diet. Specially prepared meals were served in a workplace cafeteria which allowed for a high degree of control over what and how much food was eaten. The experiment lasted for two years, a long time for this type of study.

Although the study was characterized by many as a contest between the low-fat and Mediterranean diets, the low-carb diet was the healthiest. The Mediterranean diet came in second, and the low-fat diet finished last. Members of the low carbohydrate group lost the most weight (12 pounds). Their heart disease biomarkers improved: Triglycerides were lower and HDL cholesterol was much higher than the other two groups—both healthy outcomes. Since these results didn't confirm the notion that reducing fat consumption would decrease weight and improve heart health, the study's results didn't receive much attention.

The Atkins Revolution

How had we gone so far astray? How had we overlooked the advantages of eating a low carbohydrate diet? As it turns out, we hadn't overlooked the low carb diet. Rather, we'd ignored its proponents.

In 1972, Robert Atkins, a cardiologist in New York City, published his seminal work, *Dr. Atkins Diet Revolution* (Atkins, 1972). Although his book became an overnight bestseller, he remained a voice in the wilderness promoting a view diametrically opposed to the hallowed national paradigm, the low-fat diet. Mainstream nutrition experts labeled Atkins a quack, called his diet a fad, and accused him of malpractice. Yet, Atkins held fast, ignored his critics, and pressed on. He enjoyed considerable popularity with his patients *because the diet worked.*

Robert Atkins was described as a hard-working dedicated man who was not particularly friendly or smooth. He was not a researcher, a businessman, or a politician. He was a physician, dedicated to working with and helping his patients. And, patients he treated! He reported seeing between 50 and 60 thousand patients between 1972 and his death in 2003. When questioned about conducting research studies, Atkins simply invited researchers or officials to review his thousands of case records.

Atkins' diet was scorned by academics and discredited by government funding officials. It was suggested that the large amount of fat recommended in the Atkins diet would be unhealthy, if not dangerous. Therefore, researchers didn't dare submit a research grant to study the Atkins approach. That is, until Eric Westman, a Duke University researcher, took Atkins up on his offer and reviewed his case files. Dr. Westman teamed up with Gary Foster, Stephen Finney, and Jeff Volek.

These researchers found that the Atkins diet with its increased fat consumption didn't make people sick. In fact, the reverse was true. Measures of cardiovascular health improved for people eating the Atkins diet. In trial after trial, virtually every indicator they could measure showed that a high-fat diet lowered the risks for heart disease and diabetes compared to the cherished low-fat diet. These measures included a rise in HDL cholesterol (good cholesterol), while triglycerides, blood pressure, and inflammation markers dropped.

Taking over where Atkins left off, researchers Westman, Phinney, and Volek authored the *New Atkins for a New You* (Westman, Phinney, & Volek, 2010). Over 50 research studies supporting their claims for the Atkins diet are cited in this book.

If Fats Aren't Making You Fat, What Is?

Let's return to the unfinished discussion of the processing of carbohydrates and fats by the body. We described the biological events after consuming a carbohydrate rich diet.

As a refresher, eating a carbohydrate-rich meal triggers the pancreas to produce insulin, the Swiss-Army knife of hormones. Insulin quickly shunts the fatty acids into fat cells and stands guard while escorting the glucose derived from the carbohydrates around the body to meet immediate energy needs.

After about three hours, insulin in the blood begins to decline and fatty acids are released from the fat cells into the bloodstream where they are used for energy over the long term (e.g., overnight). However, when the insulin level in our blood is elevated, our fat cells are sealed preventing the burning of fatty acids.

This was another surprising fact about fat cells. Not only do they multiply and have minds of their own, they are dynamic. They are storing and releasing fat (in the form of triglycerides) throughout the day.

Our carbohydrate-rich diets keep us reaching for snacks and sugary drinks frequently throughout the day and night. As we gain more weight, our bodies require more energy just to "feed the system". You can see the vicious, voracious spike-dip cycle emerging.

Although refined carbohydrates profoundly elevate insulin levels and keep fat in storage, eating proteins only moderately increases insulin. And, what about fatty foods like butter? What effect do these have on insulin release? The answer may surprise you. Absolutely no effect. Fat does not cause the storage of fat. Fat has no substantial effect on blood sugar levels, insulin secretion, or the conversion of excess glucose to body fat.

Fat does not make fat, refined carbohydrates do! The refined carb/low fat diet we've been encouraged to follow for decades has been contributing to our poor health and weight gain because of the havoc it creates by overloading our bodies with insulin.

Types of Fat

Now that we've established that fat doesn't make you fat, let's examine the types of fat and the benefits of eating fats. However, not all fats are good for you. Let's sort this out.

There are two major types of fat: Saturated and unsaturated. Saturated fats are easy to understand. The common types of saturated fats come from meats, cocoa butter, eggs, dairy, and palm oil. Unsaturated fats are more complicated. To help us keep track, look at the chart of the different types of unsaturated fat and their major sources

Unsaturated fats are further divided into monounsaturated and polyunsaturated, with polyunsaturated further divided into the Omega 6s and Omega 3s. Fats are divided based on their chemical structure and their stability when heated.

Unsaturated Fats

Monosaturated	Polyunsaturated
Olive Oil	**Omega 6**
Lard	Corn, Canola Cottonseed,
Chicken and	Soybean, Peanut,
Duck Fat	Safflower Oil
	Omega 3
	Fish Oil
	Flaxseed

Created through Chemical Processing
Hydrogenated Oils (trans fats)

When fats were denounced as evil in the 1950s, saturated fats were singled out as the primary culprit in promoting heart disease. Scrambling around for a replacement, the food industry settled on oils derived from seeds rather than animals. These vegetable oils are polyunsaturated fats that are pressed from seeds—cottonseed, corn, soybean, safflower, peanut, and canola. The oil in these seeds contains Omega 6s. A hydrogenation process transforms the liquid oil into a solid fat such as shortening (e.g., Crisco). In the 1960s, manufacturers shifted into high gear turning out new products containing high amounts of polyunsaturated oils including salad dressings, mayonnaise, and margarine. The Mazola oil manufacturer enthusiastically and erroneously advertised the potential health benefits of its oil by suggesting it was a medical product.

The resulting products of the hydrogenation process are known as trans fats. Trans fats are not healthy, but it took decades before this truth was made public. In the interim, we all ate these products thinking well of ourselves because we had replaced the evil saturated fats our grandparents had used.

As early as 1968, the American Heart Association (AHA) became aware of possible problems with hydrogenated oils. They initially tried to do the right thing by developing a warning brochure entitled *Diet and Heart Disease*. The booklet contained a warning.

"Partial hydrogenation of polyunsaturated fats results in the formation of trans forms which are less effective in lowering cholesterol concentration. It should be noted that many currently available shortenings and margarines are partially hydrogenated and may contain little polyunsaturated fat of the natural form."

Before thousands of pamphlets containing this warning were distributed, the AHA succumbed to financial pressures from the shortening producing industry. They revised the brochure and omitted the warning statement.

Decades would pass before trans fats were officially identified as hazardous to your health. Finally, in 1990, fresh research emerged that rattled both the scientific community and the public. The study, published in the *New England Journal of Medicine*, was a well-designed study in which a group of healthy adults were placed on a series of three different diets. The diets were identical except for fat proportion: One high in monounsaturated fats, one high in saturated fats, and one high in trans fats. During the trans fat phase, LDL rose significantly while HDL dropped significantly. This is the most unfavorable profile for heart disease prevention.

Government officials and nutritional experts ignored or minimized the study's findings. In fact, in the publication of the 1992 food pyramid, *trans fats* weren't mentioned or given the potential health hazard warning they deserved. Rather, the old warning was given: Limit saturated fats to less than 10% of total calories. Worse yet, consumers were advised to tilt their fat choices towards margarines with vegetable oil, effectively steering Americans toward some of the richest sources of trans fats and Omega 6 oils in the market.

The highly toxic trans fats were looked on fondly by the food industry because their solid form was much easier to use in baking. Seeing the writing on the wall, numerous food industry giants set about the task of removing trans fats from their cooking oils. To grasp how hard food manufacturer's work to feed our carbohydrate addictions, read this little tale.

The Oreo cookie presented a serious headache for Nabisco. With its creamy white middle sandwiched between two chocolate cookies, the Oreo cookie, a "heritage" brand was a beloved product. Changing the Oreo would alienate customers and lower company profits. One trans free recipe melted and shattered during shipping. No reformulation worked. Facing a lawsuit and millions of angry customers, Nabisco stepped up research and developed a palm oil-based mixture to make the creamy middle more stable. Overall, Nabisco spent more than 33,000 hours and conducted 125 trials to reformulate the Oreo and get it "just right."

In 2006, the AHA finally advised Americans to cut back on the harmful trans substances. In the same year, the FDA officially mandated food manufacturers to list the trans fat content of their products on nutrition labels, leaving the consumer to deal with the chaos. Some food manufacturers did partially reduce trans fats or eliminate them altogether.

Many products still contain trans fats. Be careful when buying fried foods (including French fries), baked goods, cookies, candies, snack foods, icings, and vegetable shortenings. Most margarines have been reformulated, but if the product contains less than .5 grams of trans fats per serving, a manufacturer can claim that it's "trans free." Depending on the number of servings in a product, this can result in considerable trans fat consumption over time.

As far as we're concerned, if the ingredients list mentions partially hydrogenated, hydrogenated vegetable oil, or shortening, we drop the product and run for our lives.

Omega Fats

There are two types of unsaturated fat—monounsaturated and polyunsaturated. Monounsaturated fats, such as olive oil, provide health benefits and can be used in moderation. Polyunsaturated fats are divided into Omega 6 and Omega 3 subtypes. Polyunsaturated Omega 6 fats are of concern if used in excess because they promote inflammation in the body. Omega 3s, on the other hand, provide an anti-inflammatory benefit.

From a health perspective, evaluate the Omega 6/Omega 3 ratio. Evolutionary evidence suggests that in pre-agricultural societies, humans consumed a diet that provided a ratio of 1 to 1 of Omega 6 to Omega 3, commonly expressed as 1:1. This 1:1 ratio provided ample anti-inflammatory compounds to address health concerns. However, with the dominance of refined vegetable oils so prominent in modern Western diets, the ratio has been estimated to be closer to 15:1. To correct the imbalance, we should reduce our intake of Omega 6 rich vegetable oils and increase our consumption of Omega 3 rich oils. Omega 3 can be obtained from eating cold water fish, walnuts, flaxseed, and chia seeds. Acceptable ratios can also be found in green vegetables such as spinach and leafy lettuce.

Omega 3 oils have several health benefits. One of the most important is the impact of Omega 3 oil in early life. Getting enough Omega 3 during pregnancy and infancy is crucial for the development of the child. Omega 3 can improve eye health. Omega 3 also has several benefits for heart health which include reducing triglycerides and blood pressure and elevating HDL cholesterol. Finally, Omega 3 may provide protection against autoimmune diseases.

In summary, feel free to use saturated and monounsaturated fatty acids in moderation, and increase your Omega 3 consumption. Simultaneously, drastically reduce polyunsaturated Omega 6 oils while avoiding trans fats at all costs. This includes anything labeled as "hydrogenated", "partially hydrogenated", or "shortening." In other words, do the exact opposite of what government and industry "experts" have been telling you to do for the past 60 years.

Other Benefits from Eating Fat

Topping our list of benefits from eating fat is flavor. Almonds, avocados, salmon, olives, bacon, eggs, cheese, macadamia nuts taste good, and we love to eat them. Fatty foods such as cream, butter, olive oil, coconut oil enhance the flavor of foods.

Fat when paired with protein is satisfying and curbs carbohydrate cravings. When combined with moderate exercise, added fat in the diet produces muscle gain because of better hormonal balance. Eating the right fats promotes recovery from an exercise session.

Eating the right fats in the right amount can improve cardiovascular health. Despite warnings by health officials for decades, saturated fats do not increase blood triglyceride levels. Carbohydrates, on the other hand, elevate blood triglycerides, inflammation and plaque buildup in the arteries, and increase heart disease risks. Small, dense LDL cholesterol particles increase heart disease risk, but saturated fats have no effect on these particles. Saturated fats also raise HDL cholesterol levels which may lower your risk of heart disease.

In short, many foods that are high in saturated fats (e.g., eggs, clean meats, coconut oil) can decrease inflammation, lower circulating triglycerides, and have no effect on small LDL cholesterol particles—all factors in lowering the risk of heart disease.

Fats make up the outer, protective layer of every cell in the body. This layer is composed in part by Omega 3 fats, making the cells responsive to healthy metabolic changes and helping to lessen harmful inflammation.

Additional fat in the diet allows for more hormonal balance, particularly regarding low thyroid production. Low levels of circulating thyroid hormone are linked to weight gain and may interfere with weight loss. If you haven't had your thyroid level checked, schedule an appointment with your doctor.

Dietary fats such as those found in butter, coconut oil, and fish contain the two fatty acids, lauric and myristic acid. These fatty acids are anti-viral and anti-fungal and have been found to decrease infection rates.

Getting adequate Omega 3 and a variety of saturated fats in your diet could help improve your body's ability to lubricate the skin. Dry skin and eyes are often caused by a deficiency in fatty acids. Saturated fats play a vital role in the health of bones. For example, to effectively incorporate calcium into your skeletal structure, at least 50% of your dietary fats should be saturated.

Fat and Diet Type

We'll complete this chapter with a brief look at the place of fats in commercial diets. There are three basic macro-nutrients in foods: Carbohydrates, proteins, and fats. As seen in the illustration, diets can be compared by looking at the percent of these basic nutrients recommended by authors of familiar commercial diets. For example, the standard low-fat

American diet recommends 20% of our calories come from fats, 13% from proteins, and 67% from carbohydrates. The poster child of low-fat commercial diets is the Ornish diet. At the other end of the spectrum is the Atkins diet. The Atkins diet, as originally conceived, recommends 60% fat and 33% protein, leaving only 7% in the carbohydrate category. The Mediterranean diet's fat percentage is somewhere in the middle, but the Keto diet stresses the highest fat percentage with carbohydrates low, and protein in the middle.

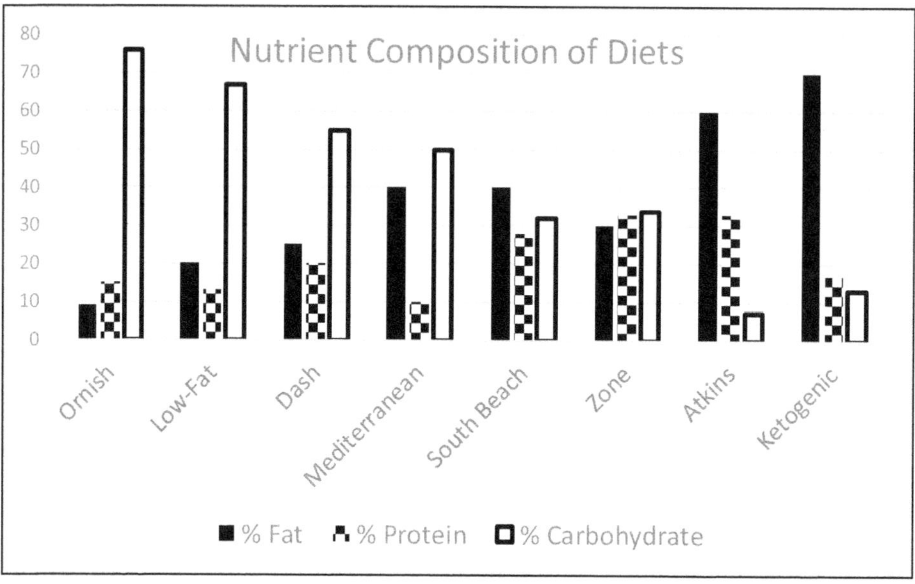

Hopefully, this chart will give you a general idea of what to look for in selecting a commercial program or, better yet, developing your own strategy.

Exercise

Select a diet book from the Internet, Barnes & Noble, or your local library. Decipher the percentage allotment of carbohydrates, proteins, and fats recommended by the author. In the next chapter, we'll take an in-depth look at proteins and fibers.

CHAPTER 9

Never eat more than you can lift. — Miss Piggy (Jim Hensen)

If I Can't Eat Carbs, What's Left?

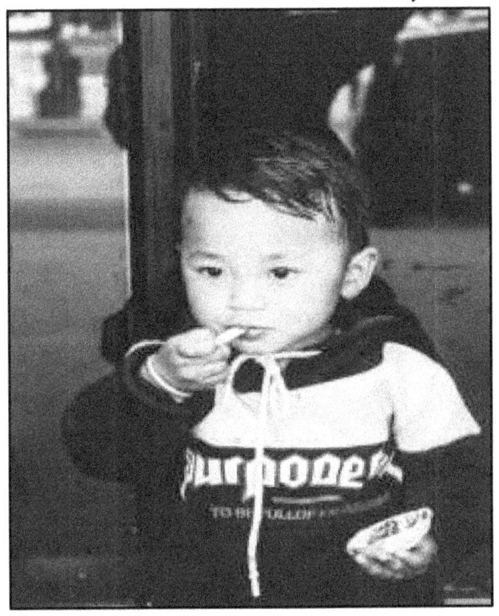

What I learned about the foods left to me after I'd given up carbohydrates was eye opening. The hardest blow was giving up fruits. I believed I could eat these with impunity. I also thought I'd been eating enough vegetables, but I hadn't. I learned to eat salad for breakfast. Our salads are now larger, richer, better, more fun, and healthier. I now eat proteins without guilt—a steak grilled in butter and slathered with sautéed mushrooms. Wow!

The photograph is by Drift Shutterbug from Pexels

* * * *

Protein is the foundational building block of a healthy body. It's so essential that without it, life isn't possible. Proteins fuel your immune system, make your hair strong, and keep your skin supple. Proteins help form the hormones, neurotransmitters, and enzymes which affect the functioning of your organs and nerves. Most important to weight loss, eating protein chases away hunger by balancing the metabolic hormones. Specifically, proteins cause your body to release hormone peptide YY which improves sensitivity to leptin, the satiety hormone. Leptin tells your brain when you are full and should stop eating. Protein also stimulates the release of glucagon which stabilizes blood sugar and prevents energy crashes—in effect, neutralizing the action of excess insulin.

The word protein comes from the Greek word "protos" which means of great importance. After water, your body is largely made up of protein. Protein is essential for the building and growth of new tissues, as well as the repair and maintenance of broken-down tissues. Tissues break down when we are physically active during strenuous work or exercise. Our bodies are constantly assembling proteins from different combinations of amino acids, each combination has a specific function determined by its amino acid sequence.

Of all the macronutrients, protein requires the most energy to digest. The breakdown of dietary protein provides amino acids. There are approximately 20 amino acids in protein, nine of which are considered essential because the body cannot make them. These amino acids must be supplied by your diet. Although people often assume that meat, eggs, and dairy products are the primary sources of protein, plant foods (e.g., vegetables, nuts, seeds, legumes, and fruits) contain some of the 20 amino acids we need. These nutrient rich plant foods can certainly complement the fish, poultry, and meats which contain all 20 amino acids.

The timing of when proteins are consumed is important. Unfortunately, many Americans have developed the habit of grab and go for breakfast, snack what's handy for lunch, and settle in for the big meal of the day in the evening. However, because of the calming and satiating action of proteins, it is important they be consumed throughout the day to counter the spiking-crashing action of insulin. Also, because of the cell rebuilding and repair process that occurs during the day, the healthier approach is to consume proteins at regular intervals. Most authorities recommend consuming a small protein snack every three to four hours. Most Americans require around 18 ounces of protein each day. It is best that protein intake be divided between, say six ounces at each meal—or better yet, nine ounces at breakfast and the remainder at lunch and dinner. This spacing of protein intake will help alleviate the 10 AM insulin crash.

The first-phase insulin responses can be modified by having some protein (meat, eggs, cheese) on hand to consume with the carbs. That is, if you slip up and inadvertently take some carb-rich no-no, eat a little protein to keep your blood glucose from rising as much as it would otherwise. The protein also helps reduce the total amount of insulin ultimately needed to handle carbohydrates and may reduce carbohydrate cravings.

Daily Recommended Amount of Protein?

Before discussing the amount of protein we need in our diet, we must consider the issue of quality. We no longer catch fish from unpolluted streams and put them on the dinner table. We rely on food producers to do the work for us. As a result, the food in our stores varies in quality. To lose weight while staying healthy, you should eat clean protein—organic plant and meat protein, fish that is wild-caught, and animals that are grass-fed and pasture-raised. The proteins from these meats are low in inflammatory Omega 6 fatty acids.

Mean proteins, on the other hand, are from animals which are grain fed and factory farmed. Protein from animals in industrial meat and dairy operations are often fed an Omega 6 rich diet of corn and soybeans. These grains make cheap feed, and the caged animals eating them fatten rapidly.

I used to think the argument for grass fed or organic protein was rubbish. How does what a cow eats and where it eats it make a difference to me? How does what the cow is fed justify the increased cost of the meat in my shopping cart? Now I know some of the answers. Products from grain-fed animals add inflammatory Omega 6 fats to our diets in a ratio of Omega 6 to Omega 3 of 8:1. Not good. By contrast, grass-fed beef has a near perfect Omega 6 to Omega 3 ratio of 1.5:1.

Also, the protein from factory farmed animals may have additional processing. Sugar, fat, and other chemicals may be added. Take your Thanksgiving turkey for example. Many of the factory farmed turkeys are injected with a saline solution and other chemicals. Processed meats high in palmitic acid, for example, may aggravate cardiovascular disease. Clearly, we need to weigh the risk of inflammation and related health problems against cost. We recommend high-quality grass-fed meats certified as organic whenever possible. High-quality animal protein is more expensive, but we believe the investment in health will pay off over the long term.

Let's turn to the issue of quantity. How much protein does our body require? There is no definitive answer to this question. In fact, there's a lot of conflicting information on the Internet, in magazines and books, and among the experts. But we'll give it our best shot.

The National Academy of Medicine recommends .36 grams of protein per pound of "ideal" body weight for adults each day. Here's an example. First, decide on your ideal weight, not your actual weight. A person weighing 220 pounds, for example, might set 190 pounds as their ideal weight. If we multiply 190 by .36, we should eat 68 grams or 17 ounces of protein each day. If we divide this by three meals, we should eat approximately 23 grams or six ounces of protein at each meal. There's a handy protein calculator on the Internet that takes several variables into account when calculating your individual daily minimum. www.proteincalculator.net

Some Protein Pitfalls

For most Americans, getting enough protein in our diet is not the problem. Most authorities agree that Americans eat too much protein. To help you assess how much protein you eat relative to carbohydrates and fats, look at the chart. Pudding has very little protein or fiber, but it has a lot of carbs. On the other end of the spectrum, a steak contains proteins and fats but virtually no carbohydrates. The sample items were taken at random from a helpful website listing the amount of fats, carbohydrates, and proteins in common foods in grams per serving. www.eatandbelean.com/fat gram food chart

It's tempting to think if a little protein is good, a lot must be better. Ahh, wrong! Although high-quality protein is crucial to good health, eating too much or choosing poor quality protein can be harmful. Our bodies simply were not designed to efficiently process large quantities of protein. Eating too much protein, even good protein, can cause oxidative stress and inflammation which contribute to cell damage (rather than cell repair). As well, too much protein can stress the kidneys and liver, the main organs concerned with cleaning up and eliminating protein waste products.

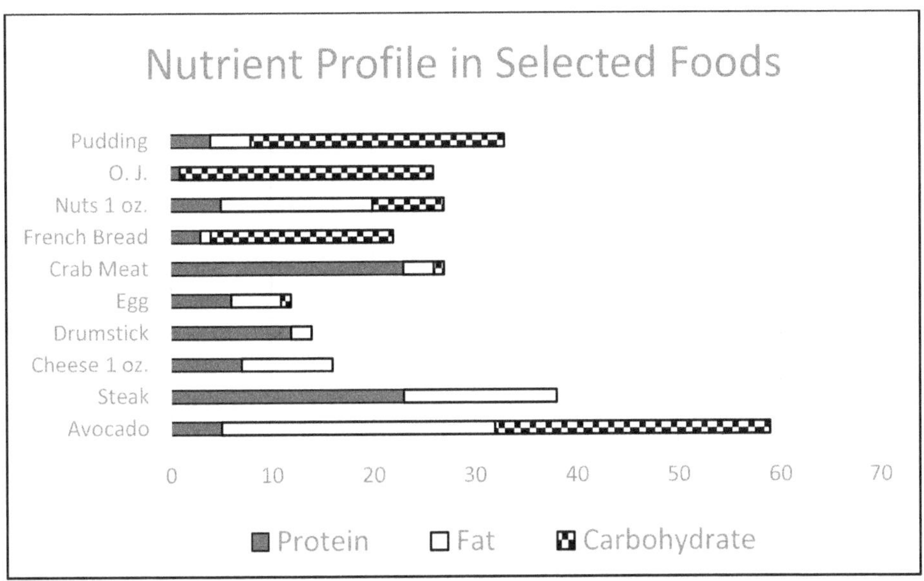

Another problem dieters encounter when consuming too much protein is stalling during weight loss—hitting a plateau you can't break. I can attest to this. I lost weight steadily for several weeks, but I hit a plateau. My weight stalled because I was eating the same amount of protein which I'd consumed during the first weeks of the diet. You will have to titrate your protein intake more than once during weight loss to continue losing. The key points are the following: 1) Eat high-quality proteins; 2) mix in plant proteins; and 3) track amount of protein and adjust total protein intake as your diet progresses.

Fructose: Sweet Danger

As most health-conscious people know, fructose is the sugar nature put in fruit. Most people think positively of and enjoy nature's candy (including L. J.). As humans evolved over the centuries, fruits were cherished as their sweet taste often indicated safety and abundance. Fruits were only eaten in season and were consumed in small amounts. To make the long story short, in days long past, humans simply didn't get much fructose. Our metabolic system never developed ways to efficiently process fructose. Because of this, eating large amounts of fructose can be problematic because of how it is metabolized by the body.

Fructose bypasses the normal glucose metabolism pathways and quickly turns to fat in the liver and abdomen. Too much fructose in our diets is associated with the development of non-alcoholic fatty liver disease (Jensen, 2018).

The fructose story makes me sad. I love fruit, but I now recognize that fruit, which I believed to be healthy in large amounts, was building my belly, Caroline.

The health issues linked to fructose were compounded by the development of high fructose corn syrup. Food manufacturers developed a way to make a fructose concentrate and combine it with corn syrup. This is a deadly combo. HFCS was added to many processed foods starting in the 1970s. With HFCS being added to every processed food from baby food to soda drinks, our consumption of fructose has skyrocketed causing near-universal metabolic chaos (insulin resistance, fatty infiltration of the liver, abdominal obesity, and diabetes). Tragically, the signs of metabolic chaos are showing up in children as young as age 10 years old.

In case you skipped over the passages related to HFCS. Read the following slowly.
Of all the food substances you and your family should avoid at all costs, high fructose corn syrup should be at the top of your list.

With fructose, moderation is the watch word. Eating a small apple or pear each day is fine. Low-fructose berries are ideal: Blueberries, raspberries, strawberries are low in fructose and contain about three grams of fiber per cup.

Fiber

We don't eat enough fiber. It is estimated that the average American consumes between 10-15 grams of fiber each day. This is about half of what we need. Shoot for 30 grams and if you consume as much as 50 grams—that's OK. fiber rich complex carbohydrates, unlike simple carbs, are highly recommended. High-fiber foods have a host of benefits. Fiber-rich foods include all forms of nutrient-dense sources such as fresh vegetables, nuts, seeds, beans, and legumes.

Like everything else in the complex world of nutrition, fiber can be defined in a variety of ways. Traditionally, fiber is divided into either dietary or functional fiber. Dietary fiber is the non-digestible woody portion of carbohydrate-based plants. Functional fiber is also a non-digestible carbohydrate that forms a gummy substance (think oatmeal). Another way to define fiber is to examine the relationship with water: whether the fiber can be dissolved in water (soluble fiber) or whether it cannot be dissolved in water (insoluble fiber).

When we cook foods that are high in water-soluble fiber, such as black beans, they break apart and begin to absorb and hold water, becoming a mushy substance. As most cooks know, when we cook water-soluble fiber foods, we need to gradually add water during the process.

Insoluble fiber does not dissolve or breakdown in water. This includes foods like celery, asparagus, brussels sprouts, broccoli, cabbage, and kale. These highly nutritious foods are also known as cruciferous vegetables. Cruciferous foods should have a prominent position in your diet.

Insoluble fiber's primary role is to regulate bowel function by aiding the movement of food through the intestines. Sources rich in insoluble fiber include whole grain products, nuts, and vegetables. Soluble fiber forms a mushy gel when digested and helps to lower cholesterol and blood sugar levels.

Many foods contain both soluble and insoluble fiber. This is because the outer layer of grains, nuts, fruits contain insoluble fiber, but the inside is soluble fiber. The outer peel of an apple or pear, for example, is composed of water insoluble fiber, but the fleshy material inside is water soluble fiber. Likewise, the outer shell of grains (so-called bran) is insoluble fiber, but the internal substance is soluble fiber. Unfortunately, in the case of grains, the outside bran is often milled off and discarded in the refining process. The internal substance is ground into white flour. This refining process is one example of how manufacturers have taken healthy food and transformed it into unhealthy food.

Eating refined foods such as white flour or white rice can result in digestive problems such as constipation. Eating insoluble fiber foods assists with regularity. However, many manufacturers of products designed to help with constipation use ingredients that include soluble fiber, i.e., psyllium. If you use one of these products, it's important to drink a lot of fluids. If you don't drink enough water, the soluble fibers can back up in the stomach and intestines.

Over time, impaction can develop in the large intestines, a very uncomfortable situation.

Excessive loss of body fluids results in diarrhea. Traditionally, the BRAT diet has been recommended for treatment of diarrhea. This diet is composed largely of bananas, rice, apples, and toast (BRAT). All these foods contain water soluble fibers. The water soluble fibers help in the absorption of excess water in the digestive system. Water soluble fibers can also make us feel full which helps with weight loss.

Most authorities advise eating a wide variety of fiber rich foods to get an adequate supply of different types of fiber in our diet. This means eating fruits and vegetables with the peel (eat the whole apple). Add lentils and black beans to casseroles and salads. Use brown rice instead of white rice and choose a high-fiber breakfast cereal (Fiber One). A cup of raspberries (8 grams) tossed on a cup of oatmeal (4 grams) gets you about halfway to your 30-gram goal.

There are several additional benefits of a high-fiber diet. These include lowering the risk of hemorrhoids, irritable bowel syndrome, and diverticular disease. An adequate amount of soluble fiber can help prevent heart disease by lowering LDL. Fiber-rich foods dampen the rise in blood sugar and help stabilize insulin levels after a meal. Fiber-rich foods decrease inflammation and lower blood pressure. Fiber-rich foods nourish healthy bacteria in your microbiome (gut) and help remove toxins from your digestive system.

Delaying the absorption of blood sugar by eating fiber helps maintain balanced glucose and insulin levels. Fiber rich foods cause the body to release insulin more gradually than it does when you eat refined junk carbohydrates. Junk carbohydrates include products which claim to contain fiber such as whole grain crackers, cereals, and chips. Unfortunately, some recent diet books steer people away from fiber rich carbohydrates in an effort to reduce overall carbohydrate consumption. We feel this is a mistake because fiber rich carbohydrates have so many benefits.

When you consume water-soluble or water-insoluble fibers to deal with digestive issues (e.g., diarrhea or constipation), make sure you work closely with your physician.
If you decide to increase your consumption of fiber, do so gradually over time. Again, work closely with your medical provider before making any changes.

Exercise

Your exercise for the week is to re-visit your pantry and look for processed foods (bottles, cans, or boxes) containing HFCS. Bet you'll find one or two. We found an old bottle of Worcestershire sauce with HFCS listed in the ingredients. Sneaky, sneaky! We understand that the makers of Advil use HFCS as a coating!

CHAPTER 10

I have never taken any exercise except sleeping and resting. —
Mark Twain

Please Tell Me I Don't Have to Exercise!

Health gurus by the legion tell us we must exercise to lose weight. Thumbs down on that. I'll tell you why. I hate exercise machines. Those shiny machines with their gears, belts, knobs, and hard little seats scare me. Maybe I'll get some important body part caught in a gear. I particularly dislike fancy exercise machines that take you on bike rides through the mountains. I'll see the Alps by auto. Thank you very much.

I hate sweating. When you exercise, you sweat. My mother would correct me here. Ladies don't sweat, they perspire. Maybe if they built exercise machines which hosed you off, I might try one.

I hate gyms. I find it intimidating to walk through a gym—all those fit bodies pounding away and concentrating ever so intently on television screens or propelling themselves to the beat of music from their iPhone. They don't look at me, but I feel their recrimination. I know what they're thinking. Lazy slob. You could look like me if you just climbed on one of these mechanical wonders. I don't like to exercise at home. It's no fun tripping over the unused exercise equipment in a dusty corner of my house. Every time I see the exercise bike sitting there gathering dust, I feel guilty. I don't like giving exercise devices away at a garage sale. It's the ultimate admission of defeat.

Is my case hopeless? Is there another way to lose weight?

* * * *

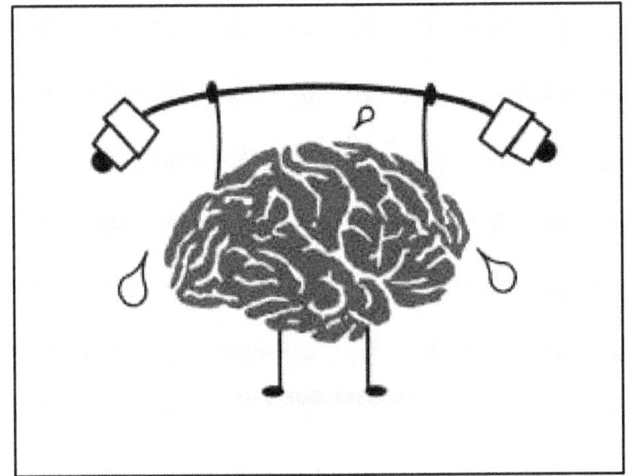

It's important to put the issue of exercise on the table early in our conversation because the myth that we must exercise to lose weight hurts us. It hinders us in our attempts to lose weight.

For the better part of the 20th century, the answer was simple and unenlightened. "Of course! You're overweight because you ate too much and didn't exercise enough." This superficially reasonable answer has one major drawback—it's not supported by science. Image by <a href="https://pixabay.com/users/Tumisu-148124/

This answer is based on a misguided interpretation of a physics postulate. Energy consumed (food eaten) must equal energy expended (exercise) or calories in = calories out. If we eat more than we exercise, we'll gain weight; if we exercise more than we eat, we'll lose.

In my past unsuccessful attempts to lose weight, I selected a plan from among the 150 on the market. My plan was based on the energy model, calories in = calories out. I counted calories, cut calories, traded calories, etc., following some mystifying system absolutely and positively designed to reduce calorie intake and make me skinny. Then came the exercise. After having not been near a gym since college, I decided to follow an exercise program that should burn off those nasty calories like a locomotive burning coal. I lived in the jogging capital of the world at the time, Eugene, Oregon. My exercise advice came from a book written by a running coach. He had a simple approach: Do this week 1, this week 2, this week 3, etc. His advice was casual and given in an off-hand manner. Exercise is simple and easy stuff. Nothin' to it. Just do it. I bought jogging shoes and a running suit and started my program.

Of course, exercising over the long term isn't easy, nor is it much fun. As you might guess, my jogging program lasted about a month or two before I started finding excuses to skip my run. "It's too rainy and cold. I'll go tomorrow." Sound familiar?

Most of us don't keep exercising, especially we folk with weight management problems. The drop-out rate for exercise programs ranges from 70 to 90%. Naturally, feelings of depression and failure set in when you stop exercising. You think you're the only one who gave up. Well, you aren't the only one. You're in the majority.

Why Doesn't Cutting Calories and Increasing Exercise Work?

High BMI, as we are repeatedly told by the media, is associated with an increased frequency of virtually every modern chronic disease. People of every age, race, gender, or national origin are told to eat less and exercise more—as if the thought of doing these things never entered our small minds. Despite near-daily reminders of severe medical consequences, well-meaning, hard-working everyday folks like you and me all around the world continue to gain weight. The experts conclude that we just didn't get the message. Let's tell them again, but louder this time. Eat less and exercise more. Well, we get the message. We just can't follow your advice.

Why do experts repeat the same advice? Mr. Banting described his miserable experience sticking with the exercise program his doctor prescribed in the 1860s. He nearly killed himself trying to follow that advice, and he didn't lose weight. Why do experts keep repeating advice that doesn't work generation after generation?

Enter the strange world of the *flawed paradigm*. A paradigm is a typical or commonly held opinion which forms the basis of a scientific subject. An example is the recommendation that we should drink eight glasses of water a day. Where did this opinion come from? It came from a one-page letter written by a physician in 1948. After that date, the recommendation was presented as if research had been done. Many times opinions are supported by evidence, but flawed paradigms such as the energy model take on a reality of their own. Once established, experts have a difficult time accepting that their paradigm might be wrong, and advice based on their paradigm is also wrong.

Why is the Energy Model Flawed?

The energy model is wrong because it is incomplete. The model ignores what scientists call intervening variables or factors. Do eating and exercise have something to do with weight gain or loss? Of course, they do. But there are many other variables which affect our weight. These have nothing to do with either eating or exercising.

The most important of these variables is our genetic makeup. Although we're not exact clones of our parents, everyone comments on a resemblance among relatives. Studies comparing the general population, siblings, fraternal twins, and identical twins show that the similarity of body type (not just facial features) increases with the genetic closeness of each group.

Another variable that messes up the energy balance model is gender and the related sex hormones. Our gender influences our shape and size. Again, common sense tells us that during the adolescent growth spurt, men grow beards, sprout an Adam's apple, and grow taller, leaner, and more muscular, while women put weight on the hips and breasts.

What about other less obvious variables. What about sleep pattern, peer group, zip code, stigmatization history? Add these in. And the list could continue, but you get the point. *The energy-model is flawed because it applies a simple solution (eat less, exercise more) to a highly complex problem (weight loss).*

What Is the Influence of Exercise?

When overweight people participate in exercise-only programs, do they lose weight? In a recent article in *Precision Nutrition*, Helen Kollias discussed a study comparing the effects of diet versus exercise on weight loss (Ball & Bolhfner, 2008). <u>https://www.precisionnutrition.com/rr-diet-exercise-weight loss</u> We liked this article by Kollias for several reasons. First, she admitted up front being a fan of exercise, an admission of bias rarely found in the nutritional literature. Second, the study used ordinary facilities (Weight Watchers, Gold Gym) rather than a university laboratory setting. Third, subjects, all female, were overweight and sedentary with a stable measured weight (i.e., previous three months). And finally, the participants were treated as members of the study, rather than patients.

In the Ball and Bolhfner study, 48 women were randomly assigned to either a weight loss diet or fitness center program. They were followed for 12 weeks. The major component of the diet program was calorie restriction, with weekly weigh-in sessions and meetings with individual counselors. The fitness group received three personal training sessions followed by a program which emphasized weight training and cardio exercises. The program followed a schedule of 30-minute sessions three times a week. Body weight, percentage of fat/lean mass, abdominal fat, and lipoproteins were assessed.

The results. Drumroll please! After 12 weeks, the diet group lost an average of nine pounds per participant, but the exercise group lost only 2.7 pounds per woman. Other studies comparing exercise to diet have reported similar results. This tells us that you might lose weight by exercising, but you won't lose much. What happens when you stop exercising? The pounds come back with a few friends.

Some studies have reported that we gain weight after heavy exercise. How could this be? A personal anecdote may have a familiar ring. R.E. used to play racquetball with a friend several times a week. After a vigorous session, they would head over to Ye Olde Pub for generous helpings of nachos smothered with cheese, salty chips, meaty pizza, etc., all washed down with frosty mugs of draft beer. And, it doesn't take many slices of pizza to exceed the number of calories burned during an exercise session. Exercise and physical exertion increase appetite. Most of us overestimate the number of calories we've burned, and we use this to justify grabbing an extra snack.

Finally, just the mention of physical exercise brings up negative feelings. Many of us were subjected to ridicule and shame in exercise settings. This ridicule may have come from an aggressive parent, a superior older sibling, a gym teacher, a commanding officer, or a bossy relative. For those of us who've experienced these humiliations, being told we should exercise rekindles these feelings of shame, humiliation, and failure. If you feel this way, trying to participate in an exercise program is doomed. No one needs more failure (Vartanian and Novak, 2011).

I'd Like to Exercise. Where Do I Begin?

We believe the best exercise program designer is you. When deciding how exercise fits in your weight loss program, keep these things in mind. Exercise has a limited impact on the amount of weight you will lose, and it may negatively impact other areas of your life (e.g., time, expense, physical pain, injury, lower self-esteem, confidence, etc.)

Because weight loss is not a benefit of exercise, exercise only because you want to, because it makes you feel good. Make sure that the positives of your exercise program offset the negative consequences in your life. If you choose exercise, you will gain the following benefits: Hormone stabilization, cardiovascular health, improved emotional state, and better sleep.

Plan your exercise program cautiously. Don't rush out and buy a four-year gym membership or fill your basement with expensive exercise machines. Make sure you have your ducks in a row. Think it through. Relax, take some deep breaths. Reflect on your past experiences with exercise. Is there something you always liked to do? Is there an activity associated with emotional trauma and abuse? Choose the former and avoid the latter.

Remember the movie *What about Bob?* Bob was an anxious and dependent man who worried about everything. His therapist told him to take baby steps. This is good advice when embarking on an exercise program.

Find a companion to exercise with. Commitment to another has two benefits. You're more likely to exercise if you have a buddy. It also increases your social contacts.

There's help available on the Internet. This includes tables of various kinds listing different exercises and activities, different time periods, and the number of calories burned. Some tables include several weight groupings. As it turns out, heavier types burn more calories than leaner types during exercise.

In sum, the answer to the question put forward at the beginning of the chapter, "Do I have to exercise?" is "Only if you want." However, if you struggle with the mere thought of exercising, it would be best to put the idea aside for now. If you set up a program and don't follow through, don't beat yourself up. Remember you're in the majority. Most of us stop exercising!

The focus in this book is on weight loss and addiction management. Exercise is only one small arrow in your quiver in the battle against carbohydrate addiction. I lost nearly one third of my body weight using diet alone. I didn't put toe one in the gym or start exercising until I had my weight under control.

Exercises

1. Read William Bantings (1863) pamphlet on his struggles to lose 46 pounds. Over a century ago, his doctor told him to exercise to get rid of his excess pounds. Exercise didn't work then, and it doesn't work now.
   https://onlinelibray.wiley.com/doi/pdf/10.1002/j.1550-8528.1993.tb00605.x
2. List the pros and cons of exercise in your life.
3. Discuss the exercise issue with the important people in your life.
4. Decide on a program. If you can't decide on a program, you're not ready.

CHAPTER 11

Be yourself. Everyone else is already taken. — Oscar Wilde

There's Only One You

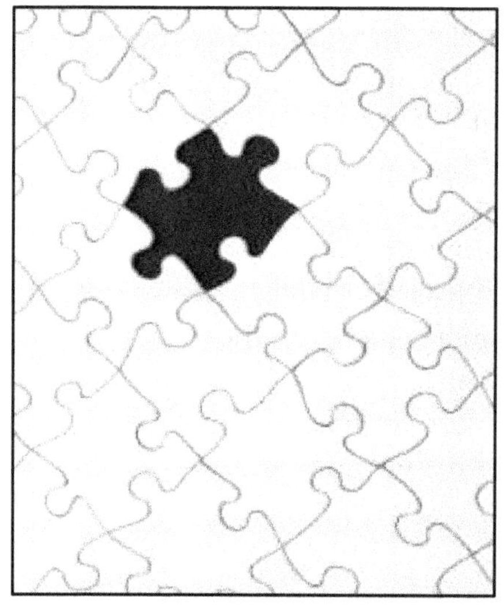

Why is Mother Nature so unkind? I know a woman who eats pie for breakfast to keep her weight up. I look at a sugar cube, and I gain weight. Why? Her genetic profile is different from mine. My profile makes me vulnerable to Carb Addiction and regaining weight after dieting. If Mother Nature weren't enough to put up with, our society emphasizes the social and personal factors involved in high BMI.

Photo www.pexels.com/photo/black-and-white-blank-challenge-connect-262488/

For some reason I can't fathom, our society does not want to believe that obesity has a genetic basis. That's despite an enormous body of scientific evidence showing that our genetic makeups are related to our weight. This evidence has been described as "unassailable" (Friedman, 2004; O'Rahilly & Farooqi, 2008). So, why worry about your genes? Your genetic makeup sets the boundaries of your weight and your ability to lose weight.

*** * * ***

There's little serious doubt that "the single most powerful determinant of inter-individual differences in adiposity (fat) is heredity" (Friedman, 2004). In other words, struggles with our weight can stem from our genetic makeup. Evidence for this comes from several sources.

There are defects in specific genes which cause monogenic (single gene) forms of overweight. (Note: Defect means that a gene pair is missing or altered.) Some of the single gene defects make us feel hungry and eat too much.

Prader-Willi Syndrome, for example, is a well-known genetic disorder. Beginning in childhood, the affected person is constantly hungry, and this usually leads to obesity followed by Type II Diabetes. There are also associated physical characteristics, mild to moderate intellectual impairment, and behavioral problems.

Additional evidence for an association between BMI and our genetic makeup comes from twin studies (Stunkard, Foch, & Hrubec, 1986; Stunkard, Harris, Pedersen, & McClearn, 1990). In a comprehensive study of identical (same genetic makeup) and fraternal twins (different genetic makeup) reared by biologically different families, researchers compared the twins' weights with those of their natural and adoptive parents. The weights of the genetically identical separated twins were remarkably similar, but their weights did not correlate with those of their adoptive parents. Remember, most of these twin pairs had no contact with their biological parents after infancy. Wardle et al. studied 5,000 11-year old twins. They estimated that the heritability of both BMI and waist circumference was high (77%). The environment in which we're raised doesn't override our genetic makeup.

Our BMI levels are linked to our parents' weights. That is, we inherit our weight gain propensities from our parents. A child's risk of having a high BMI is increased 2 ½ to four times if one parent has a high BMI and is ten times higher if both parents have a high BMI (Hinney, Vogel, & Hebebrand, 2010). My mother struggled with her weight, but my father was lean. My risk falls somewhere in the middle of the population.

Our sex also affects our risk of high BMI. If you're female, you have a higher risk of developing morbid obesity than a male. Take, for example, carriers of the MC4R gene pattern. This gene pattern is linked to a high BMI in both men and women; however, the effect of the mutation on eating patterns and weight is twice as strong for females. In a study of chromosomal locations, seven out of 14 chromosomal locations linked to high BMI were associated with waist to hip ratio. All seven of these locations showed a stronger effect on women than men.

Finally, our ethnicity affects our weight-gain risk. We put together a few ethnicity studies in the following table. The table shows the percentage of a given population which were defined by researchers as obese (Kumar, 2006; Lin et al., 2017; Wang et al., 2017). Note that Asian Americans have the best chance of remaining lean. In the United States samples, the incidence of high BMI by ethnicity in descending order is the following: African American, Hispanic, Native American, Caucasian, and Asian American.

Race	Percent
Caucasian	22–38
African American	34–47
Hispanic	28–47
Native American	34
Pacific Islanders	33
Asian American	3–13
Turks	51
Samoans	53

Samoa is dealing with a worsening health crisis. Many Samoan islanders are disabled due to the health complications of high BMI. A recent genome wide association study found a unique genetic variation not seen in other populations. It is likely that this genetic variation explains the extremely high prevalence of obesity in Samoa (Stryjecki, Alyass, & Meyre, 2018).

What about environmental factors such as diet? Can't diet explain the differences among the ethnic groups? Genetic admixture studies demonstrate that the differences between the ethnicities cannot be completely explained by diet. An admixture study analyzes an individual's genetic makeup (how much of each racial characteristic an individual has) and compares this with BMI and other indicators. For example, an African American with a greater admixture of European Caucasian has a lowered risk of high BMI than one with a smaller mixture. If income, education, and other variables are controlled, those with a higher admixture of European Caucasian have a lowered risk of obesity.

The Genetic Deck May Be Stacked Against You.

We hate to take you back to feedback loops but understanding feedback loops (homeostasis) and genetic mutations is essential to your understanding of your weight and why it is so difficult to lose weight. Most importantly, this information might help you grasp why you regain the weight you've lost.

Recall the feedback loops in the brain's reward system which tell us to search for certain foods. There are also feedback loops between the central nervous system and our digestive system which control both short-term and long-term eating (Konturek et al., 2005). The short-term loops prevent overeating during a meal, and long-term loops regulate the energy stores of our body fat.

The system which controls eating is homeostatic—it has a set point for energy use and consumption. Think of the thermostat on your heating system. You set the thermostat to the level you want, and the thermostat senses when the air temperature has gone too low or high. When either happens, the furnace or air conditioner runs until the air temperature is returned to the desired level.

Normal control of eating requires a healthy hypothalamus. The hypothalamus is the eating control center. See the diagram. The functions of the hypothalamus are similar in all mammals. The hypothalamus is a small structure situated above the pituitary or master gland. The arcuate nucleus of the hypothalamus is the control center for hunger and satiety (feeling full). The arcuate nucleus contains two distinct subsets of neurons controlling food intake. One acts as a stimulus for feeding. The lateral hypothalamic region is often called the hunger center. The neurons in this region contain neuropeptide Y (NPY) and agouti-related peptide (AgRP). The products of these neurons stimulate food intake when injected into the central nervous system (Druce, Small, & Bloom, 2004; Reinehr, Kleber, et al., 2009; Reinehr, Schmidt, et al., 2009).

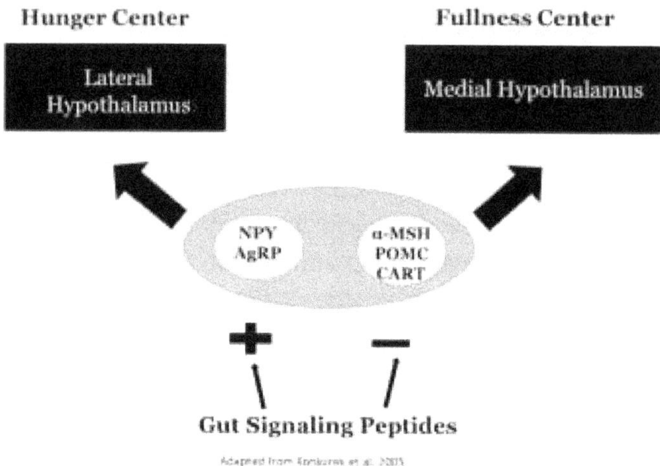

Adapted from Konturek et al. 2005

Activity in the second subset of neurons in the ventromedial hypothalamus decreases hunger, appetite, and eating. The ventromedial hypothalamus is often called the satiety center (i.e., makes you feel full.). These neurons contain α-MSH, cocaine-amphetamine-regulated transcript (CART), MR4C, and POMC. Direct administration of these compounds into the circulation of the central nervous system inhibits food intake.

The arcuate nucleus of the hypothalamus gets chemical information from the digestive organs. The digestive system produces peptides (gut stimulating peptides in figure) and releases them into the bloodstream. If peptides related to starting or stopping eating are introduced into the circulatory system of the brain, both rats and man increase their food intake, gain weight, and increase their fat deposits (Konturek et al., 2005). The receptors in the arcuate nucleus react to the circulating gut stimulating peptides and relay information to the hypothalamus activating either hunger or cessation of appetite.

For a good video describing this process, visit the Khan Academy on YouTube. They have a three-minute video entitled, *Hunger Control.*

We'll start with the primary gut or appetite-stimulating hormone, ghrelin (growth hormone releasing peptide), shown in diagram as gut stimulating peptide +. Ghrelin has been called the hunger hormone. Ghrelin is principally secreted by the endocrine cells of the stomach lining (Austin and Marks, 2009). Ghrelin levels in your blood stream increase prior to meals and then fall quickly *after* you've eaten. If you are given a dose of ghrelin before eating a buffet meal, you will gobble down 28% more than you usually do.

In contrast to ghrelin which stimulates hunger, there are many gut peptides that are associated with the sensation of fullness. All these substances reduce the amount rats eat at one feeding (insulin, leptin, choleystokinin, peptide YY, pancreatic polypeptide, incretins, glucose -dependent insulotropic polypeptide, adiponectin).

Leptin is an adipocyte hormone produced by the white and brown fat cells. Its bloodstream concentration is proportional to body fat mass, and it is known to inhibit hunger. Unlike ghrelin, leptin levels are not related to the meal pattern. Leptin levels in the blood vary with the amount of fat in the body. Leptin levels have a rhythm, and they are high between midnight and early morning and drop to their lowest point around noon.

Leptin-deficient mice and men don't have enough leptin in their bloodstream, and as a result, they become very fat. They eat too much and move too little. If they get doses of leptin, they eat less and lose weight. Some of us are leptin deficient.

About 5 out of every 100 people with high BMI are leptin deficient. One writer wrote, "It is possible that these individuals could benefit from leptin therapy" (Reinehr, Kleber, & Toschke, 2009; Reinehr, Schmidt, Toschke, & Andler, 2009). Are you one of them?

PPY is a peptide produced by the gut and released into circulation after meals. Peripheral administration of PPY decreases appetite and inhibits food intake. GRP-1, produced by the gut, is a potent inhibitor of food intake when it is administered to rats (Choquet & Meyre, 2011).

As noted earlier, insulin also reduces hunger. Insulin levels in our blood increase rapidly after a meal. After insulin enters the brain, appetite is suppressed. Mice with a neuron specific disruption of the insulin receptor gene have increased food intake and increased body fat. Insulin is important in carbohydrate addiction and is discussed in more detail elsewhere.

Genes Underlying High BMI

For most of us, our high BMI is linked to more than one gene (polygenic). Increasingly, new measurement techniques are identifying genes which are linked to high BMI. In 2001, six genes were linked to monogenic human obesity. By 2008, progress in the field led to the discovery of eight monogenic genes (FTO, PCSK1, MC4R, CTNNBL1). Genome-wide association studies led to further breakthroughs in gene identification, and now nine loci are recognized to be involved in Mendelian forms of obesity along with 58 loci contributing to polygenic obesity. We'll look at three of these.

One of the most common autosomal, monogenic (not on a sex chromosome, single gene) genetic disorders in man involves the MC4R availability. This genetic abnormality causes high BMI. It is a distinct inherited obesity syndrome (Alharbi, et al., 2007). MC4R has a central role in the control of eating (Qi, Kraft, Hunter, & Hu, 2008). Overeating is linked to a mutation in the MC4R (melanocortin-4) receptor, and it works by decreasing the available MC4R. This changes your fullness or satiety threshold (Syrjecki et al., 2018). If you have this mutation, your body doesn't tell you when you're full. This is not a rare defect.!

Out of every 1,000 persons with high BMI, one will have a MC4R deficiency (O'Rahilly and Farooqi, 2008). Are you the one person in a thousand?

A genetic variant of FTO has the highest association with high BMI thus far identified (Cecil, Tavendale, Watt, Hetherington, & Palmer, 2008). It is a causal gene underlying obesity. Overexpression of the FTO in mice increases food intake and results in obesity. FTO is associated with increased feelings of hunger in children and adults, and it plays a role in the food choices we make. Individuals with this obesity risk factor snack more, and they eat more high energy foods (Choquet and Meyre, 2011).

A congenital deficiency in proopiomelanocortin (POMC) results in a syndrome of hypoadrenalism, severe obesity, and altered hair and skin pigmentation (Farooqi et al., 2006). One copy of the POMC gene can set us up to gain weight. Genetic variations of this gene have subtle effects on POMC expression and may influence our risk of becoming overweight.

The Sticky Thermostat

Earlier we used the thermostat as an example of the homeostatic control of hunger. We can only wish that our brains controlled our appetites as well as our thermostats control temperature. Your thermostat works just as well if the room temperature is too low or too high. Sadly, our hunger control system is sticky down. In other words, your brain is set to gain weight and store fat, but it is reluctant to part with the fat it has stored.

Our bodies are tuned toward weight gain (Druce et al., 2004). Our brain sets up a standard for food metabolism, and it maintains that set point despite day-to-day variations in intake and energy use. In fact, there are few biological mechanisms which encourage weight loss, but there are strong mechanisms spurring weight gain. Take the antagonists ghrelin and leptin, for example. The effects of ghrelin (+) on appetite are much stronger than the effects of leptin (-). Eating should shut down ghrelin; but as we gain weight, this is less and less true. Eating should trigger leptin to tell us that we have lots of energy in our fat cells, but weight gain makes us less sensitive to the effects of leptin. This sets up a voracious cycle which worsens as weight gain continues. Eating now begets eating. As Nora Volkow suggested in an interview, the eating control system's brakes are shot.

Even when we lose weight, our bodies seem to remember how we used to eat. Our bodies seem to yearn to return to the past. After gastric and intestinal bypass surgery, many patients do experience long-lasting weight loss. The brief period of nutrient malabsorption passes. Yet, patients fight feelings of hunger for years after the surgery. The ghrelin levels do not return to normal, and the expected ghrelin peak before eating is not seen.

How do we explain these findings? It has been suggested that our hunger regulation system evolved during thousands of years to cope with insufficient energy supply. This probably worked well for the caveman. Better store up fat when food is plentiful in preparation for times when food is scarce. Our ancestors didn't live in a world with a super-abundant food supply. They didn't have to worry about burning off the excess calories. We, unhappily, do have to worry about excess calories, increasing numbers of fats cells, and unwanted pounds.

Summary

The information in the chapter is a bit of a cautionary tale. Hopefully, you learned the following: 1) Losing weight and keeping it off will be challenging; 2) the more weight you've gained, the more challenging the journey; and 3) your body will fight you every step of the way.

We know this might be a bit depressing but hang on. There are many reasons to be hopeful. First, if you know your genetic predisposition for high BMI is strong, set realistic goals—ones you can achieve. Many diets fail due to fantasy. You imagine yourself in a bikini, size 2, or with six pack abs. If you set your goals too high, you will set yourself up for failure. Vow to be healthy and happy and to lose the pounds you can.

Second, find comfort in the fact that there is only one you. Physicians, and to a lesser degree, scientists, study illness not health. They rely on group studies which don't necessarily apply to you. So, you can't believe everything you read in the newspaper. Be discriminating about who you listen to. You are unique, and you *can* find a path that works for you.

Third, seek help in ruling out significant genetic variations. For example, are you leptin deficient? How about genetic variations associated with FTO and MC4R? Many individuals who seek genetic counseling find the experience rewarding. For some, genetic counseling helps reduce guilt and shame (Conradt, 2009).

Finally, stop blaming yourself. To some extent, you were set up by your genetic profile and an obesogenic society. Ditch the blame and guilt. Getting rid of your sense of shame will help you lose weight. We'll learn why in the next chapter.

Exercises

1. Think about your past weight loss relapses. Were your goals realistic given your current BMI? Plan for the long game. Maybe getting rid of 10 pounds and keeping it off should be a cause for celebration. Then, you can work on the next, the next, the next —

2. Consider talking to your doctor or counselor about treatment options including genetic counseling. Please be aware that commercial genetic testing quality varies. People report getting different results from different services. Due diligence in selecting your service is recommended.

CHAPTER 12

The happiness of most people we know is not ruined by great catastrophes or fatal errors, but by the repetition of slowly destructive little things. — Ernest Dimnet

Who Are You?

My problem with weight loss advice is the one size fits all approach. Grab a book on weight loss. Any book will do. Most books start out with statistics about the world's spiraling weight gain crisis. The authors then describe some physiology, nutrition, etc. supporting their unique approach. Then they tell you to follow their program, and all will be well. The sun will shine on your new skinny self.

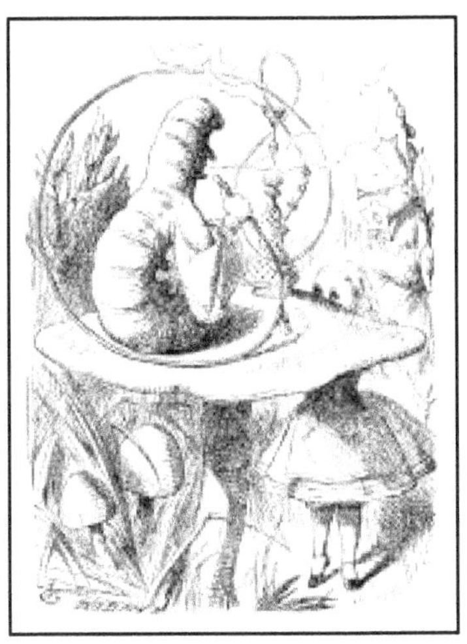

Truth is, the sun is likely to shine on your same old fat self. As we've noted, the dropout rates of diet programs are grim, about 80%. Of every 10 of us who start a weight loss program, eight of us don't lose weight. Why? We have different personalities and personal histories. Who we are determines whether we'll lose pounds or pile on pounds.

Ask yourself this question. If your cosmetologist put the same haircut on every client, would you go back? Of course, not. Should we ask less of our weight loss program?

* * * *

Like the caterpillar in *Alice in Wonderland*, we ask, "Who are you?" This may seem like a silly way to start a chapter but understanding who you are is central to losing weight. We're all products of our history and our training as well as our genetics. Our weight loss program must fit us. We can't fit the weight loss program. One researcher noted "(weight loss) programs remain for the most part unidimensional, present few options to participants, and generally cannot adapt to subjects' characteristics" (Teixeira et al., 2002; Teixeira, Going, et al., 2004; Teixeira, Palmeira, et al., 2004).

We're on your team. We want you to lose weight. More importantly, we want you to keep it off. Let's see if we can figure out who you are and why you struggle with your weight. Later we can use this information to increase your chances of losing weight (Munro, Bore, Munro, & Garg, 2011).

Tackling the emotional aspects of weight control is a giant leap into nothingness. The shortage of research on the psychological aspects of weight management surprised us. Researchers began seriously studying the impact of psychological characteristics on weight loss only recently. Given the lack of information, some might say that we're fools rushing in where angels fear to tread, but here goes.

Often scientists and medical practitioners look at the negative—what makes us sick, what makes us gain weight. After reviewing the few studies we could find on this important subject, we decided to focus on what helps you succeed (Chao, Grilo, & Sinha, 2016; Elfhag & Morey, 2008; Gerlach, Herpertz, & Loeber, 2015; Horstmann et al., 2015; Hulbert-Williams et al., 2017; James, Roe, Loken, & Rolls, 2018; Kozak, Davis, Brown, & Grabowski, 2017; Meule, 2018; Meule, Richard, & Platte, 2017; Polk, Schulte, Furman, & Gearhardt, 2017; J. Teixeira et al., 2002; VanderBroek-Stice, Stojek, Beach, vanDellen, & MacKillop, 2017; White, McKee, & O'Malley, 2007).

The beneficial personal attributes identified in these studies are listed in this table. Make a checkmark by each asset you have.

POSITIVE PERSONALITY PREDICTORS FOR WEIGHT LOSS	HAVE
No history of carbohydrate addiction	
Conscientious completer personality style	
No history of psychiatric treatment for depression	
Willing to cooperate with a counselor or advisor and have a positive relationship with counselor	
No history of emotional, physical, or sexual abuse	
Able to withstand discomfort or setbacks without giving up	
Positive body image	
No history of smoking	

The more assets you have, the less trouble you will have losing weight. In my case, I am conscientious and a task completer. I'm able to withstand discomfort and setbacks without giving up. I have no history of emotional, physical, or sexual abuse. I am satisfied with my body. I don't feel ashamed. I had smoking and alcohol dependency issues in the past, but these were in check before I started my weight loss program. I have no history of major psychiatric illness.

On the negative side of the scale, I have several challenges. I am a carbohydrate addict. I find it difficult to surrender control to others. I struggled for several weeks trying to decide whether to begin the weight loss program. I found myself wanting to reject the program before I'd tried it. I had to break down and admit that I needed help. I had to let others help me and give up my false need for control.

What's Your Style?

Will your personal style help you lose weight? You may not be sure if you are conscientious or if you're resistant to authority. To learn a little more about your style, take the Four Tendencies Quiz (Rubin, 2017). You can take the test online. This is a fun exercise to do with friends and family. You might be surprised by what you learn.

https://quiz.gretchenrubin.com/?utm_source=website&utm_medium=4Ttakequizpage

Gretchen Rubin suggests that we differ on how we balance other expectations (expectations of friends, family, and society) with inner expectations (those we place on ourselves). Based on this, she argues that people can be roughly divided into four groups: Upholders, questioners, obligers, and rebels. Upholders in her model "respond readily to both outer and inner expectations." See her book for a more comprehensive discussion of the pros and cons of each group. Questioners meet "an expectation only if they believe it's justified." In other words, they primarily respond to inner expectations. Obligers are governed by outer expectations and struggle to meet their own. Rebels "resist all expectations," both inner and outer.

Individuals who succeed in weight loss programs are generally upholders. Let's look a little more at them. They balance outer and inner expectations. They can meet the demands of others without sacrificing their own needs. They can be decisive and organized. They can take direction, and they're not rebellious.

Are you a neat freak? Do you put the spoons in the dishwasher facing the same direction? Are you teased about your tidy desk? Be glad. Laugh at those who belittle you. Your organizational bent will help you lose weight. Chances are you're an upholder. Being an upholder will help you through the diet process—fill out the food journals, take the supplements and/or medications recommended, and attend the weigh-ins and counseling sessions (Sawamoto, 2015).

Researchers don't use the term upholder. Rather they call this characteristic conscientiousness. People with high scores on conscientiousness scales are persistent and able to set and reach their goals (Elfhag & Morey, 2008).

If you are an obliger, you may not ask enough questions, and you may not share your fears and doubts. Your counselor cannot help you if you don't share your thoughts and worries.

If you are primarily a rebel and a questioner, weight loss treatment will be challenging for both you and your counselor. In my many years as a psychologist in private practice, I never failed to be amused by the client who refuted each of my suggestions. Why did the client pay me only to argue with my advice? If you have big streaks of rebel and questioner, get your questions answered before you commit to treatment. Also work through your control issues, including resistance to following the advice of others. My counselor lost 95 pounds after a lifetime of weight struggles. She knows something I don't. I finally decided to trust her. You must find someone you can trust, or your weight loss efforts won't get very far.

Body Dissatisfaction

Another important characteristic influencing weight loss success is body dissatisfaction. Unfortunately, most of us are dissatisfied to some degree with our bodies. For some of us, the level of dissatisfaction becomes phobic leading to bulimia and anorexia nervosa. We find our bodies repugnant and disgusting. For women between the ages of 40 and 60, more than 80% are trying to lose weight or maintain weight (Teixeira et al., 2002). Men have fewer problems in this area, but thanks to the bulked-up hunks displayed in the media, they're catching up. People who are very dissatisfied with their bodies lose less weight than those with a more positive attitude. Thus, hating myself because I couldn't lose weight was one factor which kept me from losing weight. Ironic, isn't it?

A behavioral model drawn from bulimia nervosa research suggests that negative self-evaluations (self-worth, body size, and shape) lead to unhealthy eating behaviors. These evaluations lead, in turn, to eating foods loaded with sugar and fat. This food combination soothes the negative feelings by stimulating the reward system (Hymowitz, Salwen, & Salis, 2017). If you eat energy dense foods (filled with fats and sugars) to soothe psychic pain, you will gain weight as surely as the night follows the day.

Now, distressed by your weight gain, you try to get your weight back under control. You may fast, purge, overuse diet pills, over exercise, etc. These are unhealthy corrective efforts, and they don't work. Failure in your frantic attempts to control your weight eventually leads to an abandonment of all dietary control efforts. Thus, a negative self-perception and poor sense of self-worth leads to disordered eating which in turn increases your risk of becoming what you most fear, being overweight.

Do you resent the ways in which your weight limits your life? Do you blame your weight for problems at work, your kids' misbehavior, your social life, etc.? If you're angry with your body, your body will hang onto all those calories. Your anger at yourself is affecting your cortisol and ghrelin levels, and this makes your body hold onto those pounds as we will see in a later section.

Distress Tolerance

Are you easily brought to tears? Do you withdraw rather than face a difficult situation? Do you get frustrated and give up when things get hard? Do people say you're thin skinned? Do you have a low pain threshold? Are you embarrassed by your inability to handle negative emotions such as anger, fear, or sadness? Do you feel guilty and ashamed about your weight? If you agree with many of these statements, you probably have low distress tolerance (Kozak et al., 2017).

Distress tolerance is a trait defined by your ability to handle negative emotional and/or physical states. If you have low distress tolerance, you probably try to avoid experiencing strong emotions like fear, pain, anger, and sadness. However, it is not always possible to avoid these feelings. Then, what do you do? What some of us do is turn to unhealthy compensatory behaviors such as drinking alcohol, smoking or overeating (or all three). These compounds light up the reward system, and we feel better, for a moment or two anyway. If you want to evaluate your distress tolerance. Take the Distress Tolerance Scale at the end of this chapter (Simons, Gaher, Oliver, Bush, & Palmer, 2005).

The Distress Tolerance Scale looks at four aspects of distress.

- Tolerance. Your evaluation of your ability to tolerate emotional distress
- Appraisal. Your evaluation of your distress
- Regulation. Your efforts to alleviate your distress
- Absorption. Amount of your attention taken by your distress

If you struggle with distress tolerance, you react strongly to negative feelings, try desperately to get out of stressful situations, suppress negative feelings, dislike your feelings of distress, and spend a lot of time thinking about negative emotional situations, you will find it difficult to lose weight and maintain your weight loss gains.

If you have a low average score on the Distress Tolerance Scale (i.e., in range 1-2), you have significant issues with managing distress. If you have a score between 4 and 5, you can manage emotional distress without going into a self-destructive and time-consuming spiral.

Take an example from my life. I worked in a difficult job with an insensitive supervisor. I resented his arbitrary and destructive decisions and his insensitive treatment of my coworkers. I spent hours describing the horrors of my situation to my very patient husband over more than a few cocktails. I couldn't handle the distress triggered by my negative emotions. Eventually, I left the job, and I since have developed better strategies for derailing this destructive process.

Impulsivity

Another personality factor which supports eating more than our body requires is impulsivity (Elfhag & Morey, 2008; Horstmann et al., 2015; Meule, de Zwaan, & Muller, 2017; VanderBroek-Stice et al., 2017). We all have a general idea what is meant by the term impulsivity. For example, the impulsive shopper buys items which are not on the grocery list. Teenage drivers are thought to be impulsive because they act without considering all the hazards on the road (unlike the rest of us).

Researchers have uncovered a new relationship between overeating and impulse control. Individuals with high BMIs are more likely to act impulsively when dealing with strong negative emotions. Impulsivity may be linked to an inability to tolerate stress and discomfort. Another facet of impulse control that relates to weight gain is preferring immediate rewards to long-term benefits. Let's look at a typical study. Lean and high BMI individuals are given a task which requires persistence. They are offered two types of reward when they complete the task. They are offered a small reward immediately after the task or a much larger reward if they choose to wait. If you have a high BMI, you're more likely to take the immediate gratification. In other words, you want to feel good in the present. The future be damned.

Another related topic is automatic eating. Have you eaten an entire bag of potato chips and felt surprised when you pulled the last chip from the bag, realizing with a jolt that you'd reached the bottom of the bag? Research has uncovered a possible mechanism. If you have a high BMI, you don't maintain your interest or attention for as long as a lean individual might. The decline in cue sensitivity or reactivity applies to what we eat and what we see or hear. However, our brains play a curious trick. They also set a low threshold for new stimulation. If there is a food ad on television and you have a high BMI, you're more likely to go to the refrigerator than the lean guy sitting next to you (Horstmann et al., 2015). What an odd puzzle. New food stuff grabs our attention, but we lose interest and switch to autopilot when food is delivered.

You can see why being impulsive interferes with efforts to lose your weight. You must persist to lose weight, you must withstand the physical challenges which accompany major changes in your eating pattern, and you must value future rewards more than present comfort.

To Smoke or Not to Smoke

If you struggle with weight gain, you may also struggle with controlling other impulses. This one is tough to face but assess yourself honestly. Many people who are addicted to carbohydrates are also addicted to cigarettes (Chao, White, Grilo, & Sinha, 2017). Cigarette smoking increases your consumption of high-fat foods, fast foods, and junk foods. We all know eating too many high-fat foods will load on the pounds. Also, smoking changes the sensitivity of the receptors in your tongue. This change may explain a smoker's preference for high-fat foods.

Many individuals with both carbohydrate and smoking addictions believe that stopping smoking will make them gain weight. This is what we thought before researching this book. Smokers weigh, on average, only slightly less than non-smokers. Our naïve belief that stopping smoking will make us fat is magical thinking. Smokers and non-smokers both lose weight in diet programs, and there is no difference in their success rates. The bottom line is this. Don't let your nicotine addiction keep you from starting a weight loss program.

Smoking not only alters your risk for several nasty diseases, but it also changes your fat distribution. Smoking promotes fat accumulation in the belly and viscera. If you're like me, it's the belly fat you want to get off. Smoking interferes with our ability to get rid of belly fat.

Should you quit smoking? This is a very tough question for us. We see two sides to this issue. One side is the risk of tackling two addictions at the same time. Should you try to beat smoking and carbs? On the other side is the way in which smoking causes an unhealthy fat distribution. Smoking may make it more difficult to pull fat from your viscera.

Which is the more important? We wish we had an answer, but we don't. We know that you're more likely to drop out of a weight loss program if you smoke. We can give you this general advice. Look at the severity of your addiction to cigarettes versus carbohydrates. If you're a heavy smoker and have a very high BMI, tackle one vice at a time. Start with food. You have a better chance at changing your eating pattern. If you have a mild nicotine dependency, tackle it before trying to lose weight.

Abuse Makes Stress and Stress Makes Fat

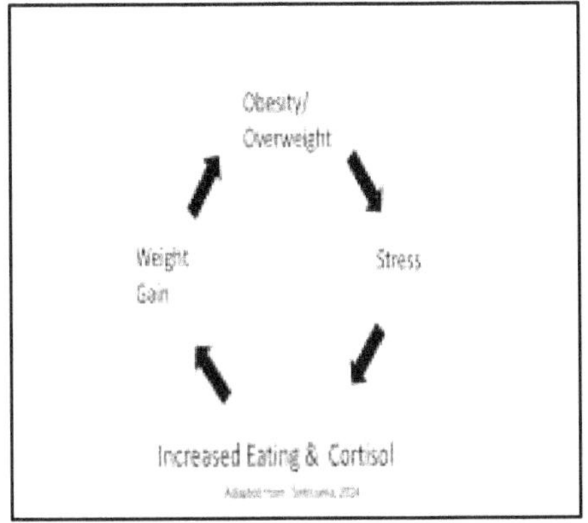

The research model of Janet Tomiyama can help us makes sense of these important psychological or personality factors. We'll cover the evidence for the model in a later chapter. She proposed this sequence of events: Shame causes stress, stress causes the hypothalamic-pituitary axis (HPA) to stimulate the adrenal gland, and the adrenal gland pumps out more cortisol to help us meet the crisis, etc. The cortisol makes us hungry, and we eat more. That causes more stress, and around we go (Tomiyama, 2014).

We're going to add an additional feature to the model. Childhood abuse triggers chronic stress which puts the HPA axis on high alert even when threats are mild or inconsequential. The chronic stress produces a lasting or chronic dysregulation of the HPA axis. Some describe this process as changing the body's set point (Hemmingsson, 2018). In other words, the body's processes for regulating energy homeostasis are permanently altered by chronic high stress. It's as if the body were telling us, "Get ready. Better load up on some sugar mixed with a ton of butter. Something bad could happen at any moment."

Chronic stress has a striking impact on your body's fat storage. Chronic stress increases the fat mass, and the fat distribution is shifted from the legs and arms to the abdomen and viscera (supposedly protects vulnerable organs from traumatic injury). We call this the skinny-legs-big-belly syndrome.

There is a critical period for developing life-long weight problems. In biology, a critical period is a developmental window in which certain events can occur. After the window closes, the developmental event cannot occur. For weight gain, the critical period is between birth to age five (Hemmingsson, 2018). In general, the severity and number of abuse events is related to later problems regulating weight. Abuse during the critical period sets up a body and brain imbalance which follows us throughout life.

Oprah Winfrey, an extraordinary survivor of sexual, emotional, and physical abuse, has discussed her life-long struggles with her weight. Her weight has varied from 125 pounds to the mid-200s, and she has lost and regained weight several times. She has also shared her history of emotional, physical, and sexual abuse. In an interview with David Letterman, Oprah discussed some of the childhood abuses. She reported that her grandmother beat her regularly. She described one sequence of beatings. "I went to the well to get some water and carried it in a bucket. And I was playing in the water with my fingers, and my grandmother had seen me out the window and she didn't like it. She whipped me so badly that I had welts on my back and the welts would bleed. And then when I put on my Sunday dress, I was bleeding from the welts. And then she was very upset with me because I got blood on the dress. So, then I got another whipping for getting blood on the dress."

At age 6, Oprah moved in with her mother. At age 9, she was raped. After the rape, the rapist "took me to an ice cream shop—blood still running down my leg—and bought me ice cream." She was sexually abused until age 14. When she became pregnant and a detention home wouldn't admit her, her mother said, "You are getting your ass out of this house."

Physical and sexual abuse in childhood creates a condition of chronic stress which in turn increases the individual's risk of becoming obese as an adult (Aaron & Hughes, 2007; Hemmingsson, 2018; Hemmingsson, Johansson, & Reynisdottir, 2014; Hymowitz et al., 2017; Mossle, Kliem, Lohmann, Bergmann, & Baier, 2017; Noll, Zeller, Trickett, & Putnam, 2007; Pinhas-Hamiel, Modan-Moses, Herman-Raz, & Reichman, 2009; Richardson, Dietz, & Gordon-Larsen, 2014). Individuals who experience physical abuse, for example, have a 33% higher probability of becoming obese as adults compared to individuals who didn't experience physical abuse in childhood (Aaron & Hughes, 2007; Mossle et al., 2017).

In a national study of United States adolescents who were followed for 13 years into adulthood, there was an increased risk of obesity in sexually and physically abused teens (Richardson et al., 2014). In another prospective study, 42% of abused adolescents became overweight as adults. When the rate of weight increase is examined, abused children have a steeper rate of weight gain or biomass increase than those who were not abused. Thus, with each passing year, the abused children's weight problems worsened (Noll et al., 2007).

You might think these statistics don't apply to you. You weren't beaten until you bled, and you weren't raped. As it turns out, emotional abuse also takes its toll. "Emotional abuse uniquely and significantly predicts disordered eating attitudes and behavior" (Hymowitz et al., 2017). It is extremely damaging to grow up with parents who minimize and ignore your emotions (Sawamoto, 2015). Both physical abuse and emotional neglect trigger a condition of chronic stress and set us up to find comfort in highly processed, energy dense foods.

You might also think that the effects of emotional abuse end when you leave the situation. Oprah Winfrey is a billionaire, but she carries the abuse in her body. In one study, emotional abuse predicted binge eating five years later (Hymowitz et al., 2017). Although our minds may trick us into believing we've left the abuse behind, our bodies remember.

Because our bodies won't forget the abuses of the past, it is difficult to lose weight. It has been established that individuals with an abuse history find it more difficult to lose weight. Why? We form junk food self-medication habits and become either fully or subtly addicted. Hemmingsson (2018) suggests the following: "Once stress, insecurity and emotional turmoil have been established at an early age, the individual will naturally seek relief from these uncomfortable states, with little interference from cognitive processes, through the brain-reward system." Junk foods, which have an exaggerated energy density through processing and food additives, are rewarding and pleasurable. We self-medicate our uncomfortable feelings with junk food. Hymowitz and colleagues (2017) call this "stress eating". Regular eating of junk food to alleviate stress changes the way the brain looks at food. You can't wish or think these brain changes away.

We're sorry to say this, but weight loss programs, dietitians, counselors, physicians, and bariatric surgeons often don't consider our emotional histories when laying out a weight management intervention (Hymowitz et al., 2017). We are left to figure this out for ourselves. This isn't good enough.

We must bring up our emotional challenges with our weight loss providers. The way in which we address these challenges is pivotal to our success. We must ask our providers to help us find ways to undo the brain-pain-food connection. Sometimes, the client must educate the provider.

A brief word about diagnosed psychiatric illness. If you have a history of depression treated with antidepressant medications, you face two additional challenges. First, depression makes you less likely to complete a weight management program. Weight loss is hard enough without piling on a mood disorder. Second, one major side effect of many psychotropic medications is weight gain. Discuss your psychiatric history with your weight loss provider. Together you can find ways to overcome these challenges.

Exercises

1. What are your personality assets? What are the good qualities that you bring to a weight loss program?
2. What are your personal challenges? Can you think of ways to manage these challenges?
3. Write the story of emotional and/or physical abuse in your life. If you don't like writing, tell your story to someone. Do you believe your body is in a state of chronic stress? Are there any stressors you can control or eliminate?

DISTRESS TOLERANCE SCALE (SIMON AND GAHER, 2005)

Directions: Think of times that you feel distressed or upset. Select the item from the menu that best describes your beliefs about feeling distressed or upset. If you strongly agree with the statement, score as follows:

1. Strongly agree (Mark 1 as your answer.)
2. Mildly agree (Mark 2 by your answer.)
3. Agree and disagree equally (Mark 3 as your answer.)
4. Mildly disagree (Mark 4 as your answer.)
5. Strongly disagree (Mark 5 as your answer.)
   ANSWER ALL ITEMS

1. Feeling distressed or upset is unbearable to me. _____
2. When I feel distressed or upset, all I can think about is how bad I feel. _____
3. I can't handle feeling distressed or upset. _____
4. My feelings of distress are so intense that they completely take me over. _____
5. There's nothing worse than feeling distressed or upset. _____
6. I can't tolerate being distressed or upset as much as other people. _____
7. My feelings of being distressed or upset are unacceptable. _____
8. I'll do anything to avoid being distressed or upset. _____
9. Others seem to be able to tolerate being distressed or upset more than I can. _____
10. Being distressed or upset is a major ordeal for me. _____
11. I'm ashamed of myself when I feel distressed or upset. _____
12. My feelings of being distressed or upset scare me. _____
13. I'll do anything to stop feeling distressed or upset. _____
14. When I feel distressed or upset, I must do something about it immediately. _____
15. When I feel distressed or upset, I cannot help but concentrate on how bad the distress actually feels. _____

Total = _______ Add scores for 15 items; then, divide this total by 15.

If you have an average score of 1, you have difficulty tolerating uncomfortable situations. If you have an average score of 5, you are more resilient.

CHAPTER 13

I think I'm still looking for a man who could excite me as much as a baked potato. — From the movie Eating

I Don't Want to Crave Ice Cream. I Can't Stop Myself. Why?

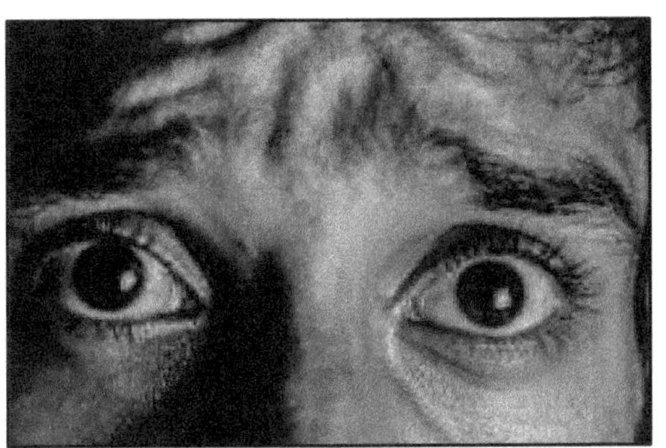

Somehow, we want to believe that understanding why eating a tub of ice cream is bad for us will make us change our behavior. In general, teaching nutritional knowledge and awareness doesn't change how or what we eat (Myers, 2015). Also, we don't want to accept that overeating is an addiction, not a simple matter of choice. Carbohydrate addiction must be managed like other addictions. It's time for the debate about whether carbohydrates are addictive to end. We must bring our knowledge about substance abuse into the management of carbohydrate addiction. A major hurdle for all addicts, including carbohydrate addicts, is managing those nagging cravings. Photo by Samer Daboul from Pexels

* * * *

Remember the Yale Food Addiction Scale. If you didn't take the scale, take it now. If you're a carbohydrate addict like me, there are things you can do to manage your addiction. Note that we don't say you can cure your carbohydrate addiction. Addictions cannot be cured—only managed. There's a large and important literature on the effects of drugs on the reward system. There are many treatment interventions designed for substance abusers that will be applied to the treatment of eating disorders. However, much of this lies in the future. We need to manage our carb addiction now, not later. We'll set down a few rules derived from substance abuse research and make several suggestions which we hope will help you cope with the upsets of life without carbohydrates.

It's no coincidence that the increase in the BMIs of people in the United States has paralleled the number and variety of processed foods on our grocery store shelves and the number of fast-food restaurants. It wasn't that long ago (1955) that McDonalds opened its first fast-food franchise in Des Plaines, Illinois. Going to McDonalds for a burger was a treat, an exciting expedition. Now, entire strip malls are lined with fast-food restaurants. Our grocery stores are at least four times the size they once were. Most of the additional space was added to answer our demand for highly processed foods.

To develop a good craving intervention plan, you need to take a hard look at the types of foods you eat. Do you eat highly processed foods such as pizza, ice cream, cake, or cookies? Yes, these are the foods in boxes, cans, and cartons. Highly processed foods contain a combination of sugars and fats which are more potent together than individually. Relative to these highly processed foods, how many minimally processed foods do you eat? Minimally processed foods are in their natural form and include nuts, fruits, vegetables, meat/fish, and some healthy dairy (high quality milk, cottage cheese, yogurt, and cheese).

If you're eating a lot of processed foods relative to foods in their natural form, you are more likely to have problematic overeating. Neuroimaging studies of the reward system in the brain suggest that pictures of highly processed foods, those foods loaded with fat laced carbohydrates, activate our reward systems. Cues linked to alcohol and drug abuse have the same effect (Polk et al., 2017). In other words, highly processed foods are addictive.

Do you find yourself thinking about the piece of chocolate filled with caramel and nuts in your pantry? Have you found it difficult to concentrate on what you're doing until you eat that chocolate? This is a description of a craving. Scientists define cravings this way. A craving is a thought driven by a strong motivation to get and eat a certain food (Joyner, Kim, & Gearhardt, 2017). Skorka-Brown et al. described cravings as "elaborated intrusions by cognitive emotional states involving embedded sensory imagery" (Skorka-Brown, Andrade, Whalley, & May, 2015).

Strong cravings usually have vivid visual images. You think of French fries, and you see them, taste them, and smell them in all their starchy glory. People report their cravings in visual (40%), olfactory (16%), and taste terms (31%). They seldom have associated sound experiences (e.g., hearing the crunch of a potato chip) or touch experiences (feel the crunch or texture of the food). Cravings are developed over time or elaborated upon by repeated pairings of sensations and emotions. These elaborated brain processes take over our consciousness.

Cravings are common. Most of us have them. Polk and colleagues asked subjects to take the Yale Food Addiction Scale and report their cravings for high- and low-processed foods (Polk et al., 2017). They had three important findings. The first was that cravings are stronger for highly processed foods than they are for minimally processed foods. We don't crave walnuts or broccoli. We crave pie, chocolate, and potato chips. Second, subjects with high scores on the carbohydrate addiction scale had stronger cravings for highly processed foods. If you scored high on the addiction scale, you are more likely to have food cravings than someone who does not score in the carbohydrate addiction range. Third, individuals with high BMI's had stronger cravings than those with lower BMIs. These results tell us that our cravings for highly processed foods increase with the amount we weigh. If we eat many highly processed foods, we want more highly processed foods. If you have very vivid or strong cravings, this means your cravings are likely to be persistent and difficult to ignore.

Cravings and Hunger

When people are asked why they abandoned a weight loss program, the most common answers are hunger and cravings. You have a better chance of long-term success if you have a plan for managing the inevitable cravings. For the more fortunate, cravings are mild and easily overcome. For others of us, cravings are why we are unable to change our eating habits and lose weight.

Cravings are triggered by many things, but the most common cause is something sensory which reminds you of the food. For example, you might hear an ice cream truck pass by, see an advertisement on television, or smell the aroma of your neighbor baking cookies. If you hear a slogan advertising a fast-food restaurant, you begin to crave a burger. The voice of a friend you often share lunch with can trigger a craving (Hoogeveen, Jolij, Ter Horst, & Lorist, 2016). I love to read mystery books, but I have trouble with authors who focus on food. A detailed description of a spectacular brunch complete with croissants sends me right to the refrigerator.

A craving can also come from a thought or a memory. Many of our food choices are made without seeing, hearing, or smelling a food. They come from our memories, both the good and the bad. We remember the wonderful Christmas dinner our grandmother always served, and we munch a few more crackers. Other times, the craving is subliminal and below our conscious awareness (Berridge & Robinson, 2016). We don't notice any change in our feelings, but we go to the refrigerator as if propelled by a mysterious unseen force.

As it happens, cravings and hunger are linked. Once a craving begins, what happens next is the activation of the brain's reward center. Your reward center pumps out some dopamine and you begin to want the sugar laced foods. Your gut reacts by making more peptides. Now you feel hungry.

The sequence of cravings to hunger will occur no matter how much or how recently you've eaten. Once again, your brain has played a nasty trick on you. It tells you that you're hungry when you have no physiological need for food.

Liking Versus Wanting or Craving

In our everyday world, liking and wanting appear to be much the same thing. If you like something, you want it—wanting and liking work in parallel. For carbohydrate addicts like us, wanting and liking are two different things. For example, consider a woman who enrolls in a weight loss program. Her mind says, "Enough, let's get this weight off. I'm going to eat healthy foods from now on," but she can't stop thinking about her favorite candy bar. She doesn't want to like candy bars anymore. She knows eating them is making her gain weight. She feels terrible when she succumbs to her craving and eats a candy bar, but she can't stop herself.

Liking and wanting are disconnected for her because she is a carbohydrate addict. When we talk about wanting, we are also talking about craving (Polk et al., 2017). The wanting or craving overrides the woman's mental determination to lose weight and avoid carbohydrates.

Let's look at how this disconnect between wanting and liking develops. The incentive sensitization theory of Robinson and Berridge (1993) has been described as the "preeminent framework in the field of addiction research" (Polk et al., 2017). This theory says that wanting (craving) motivates the use and abuse of carbohydrates more than liking or the enjoyment and pleasure derived from eating them. Why do we continue to want something we no longer like? The incentive-sensitization model suggests that liking and wanting are in harmony early in the addiction process. As the brain's reward centers are bombarded by too much sugar, drugs, or alcohol, the brain's responses to the substance or carbohydrate changes. The reward centers become hyper-reactive. Our eating of carbohydrates is now compulsive and out of control while our liking remains the same.

For example, individuals who more frequently eat ice cream have reduced responsivity in the reward regions of the brain (striatum), and their cravings for ice cream are increased (Polk et al., 2017). Liking for ice cream, however, remains the same. How often we eat certain foods can influence the relationship between craving and liking over time.

Robinson and Berridge's discovery of the incentive-sensitization principle was a fortunate accident. They placed chemical lesions in the reward centers of rats' brains. They expected to find evidence for the role of dopamine in the reward system of the brain. When researchers gave sweet substances to rats, they, like us, show facial pleasure by facial relaxation and rhythmic movements of their mouths and tongues. When given bitter tastes, the rats yawned and turned away. The researchers damaged the rats' dopamine pathways, and they expected that the rats would no longer show pleasure when they were given a sugary food. The rats continued to like the sweet taste, but they weren't motivated to eat. In other words, rats liked the sweet taste, but they no longer wanted it.

Is the same dissociation between liking and craving or wanting seen in man? The answer is "yes". The critical reader might be asking, "Is there anything I can use, or is this just an interesting theory?" The research generated by the incentive-sensitization theory has led to several important observations. These observations then led to several techniques for managing cravings.

One of the most important implications of Robinson and Berridge's work was an understanding of how persistent cravings can be even after periods of abstinence. For example, if you haven't eaten chocolate for six months, does this mean you're free of chocolate cravings. The answer, unfortunately, is "no".

We'll look at substance abuse where more is known. Overuse of a drug like alcohol or cocaine results in an enduring sensitization of the reward system. In other words, once the craving process is started, it is extremely persistent.

The drugs do not have to be "on board" for the craving process to continue (Berridge & Robinson, 2016). Cravings occur in substance abusers even though they no longer take drugs or want to take drugs. Cravings can disappear briefly only to reappear months later. The cravings sometimes return in a stronger form. The reappearance of cravings after a long period of abstinence has caused more than one relapse. Periodic issues with cravings can last for months or even years.

A second important research finding is the importance of a binge eating pattern in the control of cravings. The sensitization of the mesolimbic reward system in response to overeating of carbohydrates or overuse of drugs is stronger when there are high doses of food or drugs which are spaced apart (Berridge & Robinson, 2016). Thus, the slow steady carbohydrate overeater probably will have fewer problems with cravings than the binge eater who restrains for a few days and then eats an entire pie in a single sitting.

The third important idea from the incentive-sensitization literature is the time course of an individual craving. Your sensitized dopamine system produces pulses of dopamine release, motivation, and, finally, activation (Berridge and Robinson, 2016). These dopamine pulses are brief, lasting only seconds to minutes. If we can outwait the ordinary spontaneous craving, it may disappear. The wait-it-out strategy, however, is unreliable because some cravings are prolonged by our emotions. If we have a craving and we are depressed, the feeling will prolong the craving making it more difficult to resist.

Cues Cause Cravings

For the carbohydrate addict, the reward system, sensitized by overuse of carbohydrates, is hyper-reactive to eating-related cues. The context in which addictive foods have been eaten triggers intense wanting or craving when either encountered or imagined (Berridge and Robinson, 2016). The cues start cravings, the cravings start dopamine in the reward center, and dopamine surges start hunger.

We know that the cues-cravings-relapse cycle is true for the alcoholic or drug abuser, but we may not have considered the cycle's relationship to carbohydrate addiction. Try this brief exercise. Think of yourself as an alcoholic and consider this situation. You're invited to a celebration party at a local bar. You know everyone will be drinking alcoholic beverages. How should you manage this? Should you vow to attend but "just say no"? Should you order a non-alcoholic beer or wine so you can fit in? Should you stay home? If you think of yourself as an alcoholic, the answer is obvious and generally accepted. We all know that bars are dangerous for alcoholics. There are too many cues which will cause cravings and then relapse. Early in the recovery process, your best approach is to avoid the temptation.

Now consider a parallel situation. You're invited to a family gathering of the type described by Tomlinson—fried chicken and desserts everywhere. You're faced with the same choices—go and use your will power to refrain from eating what isn't on your diet, go and try to find something you can eat, or stay home. The answer to this quandary is less clear for carbohydrate addiction. It shouldn't be. Family meals and restaurants are the bars of the carbohydrate addict. The powerful food cues in these situations are just as dangerous for the food addict as those in a cocktail bar are for the alcoholic.

Joyner and colleagues demonstrated the power of food related cues in a naturalistic study (Joyner et al., 2017). They set up a laboratory which resembled a fast-food restaurant. Their mock restaurant offered foods often available in fast-food restaurants—French fries, milkshakes, and cheeseburgers. The foods were cooked in the laboratory before the subjects arrived, and the lab smelled like a fast-food restaurant. The mock restaurant had condiments, napkin holders, tables, and music in the background. There were menu boards with images of the foods. The lab staff were dressed in uniforms. The neutral environment had no food cues. By contrast, the foods were offered in a standard office space.

The researchers were interested in how hungry the participants were and how much they would eat in each of the environments. People in the cue-rich mock restaurant reported more feelings of hunger than those given the same foods in an office environment. The subjects also ate more in the mock restaurant. In fact, they ate significantly more. Those eating in the mock restaurant ate 220 additional calories. This number of calories is important. If you eat only 148 extra calories each day, you will gain 15 pounds per year. Eating in a cue-rich environment can lead over time to significant weight gain through small daily increases in consumption.

Controlling and Managing Cravings

Here are some suggestions for improving your chances of reaching your dietary goals by managing food cravings.

Reinterpret cravings. Don't believe that hunger or a craving means you need food. Your homeostatic mechanisms which control hunger have been corrupted by too much carbohydrate consumption. If you can't stand the hungry sensation, eat a fat or a protein instead. Small amounts of either fat or protein will blunt hunger. This technique is particularly helpful during an insulin-glucose crash.

Respect the power of cues on cravings and overeating. You are battling a powerful cue-brain-craving cycle which you've built over the years. Don't put yourself in danger until you have established some degree of control. Joyner and colleagues suggest that you avoid eating in restaurants and particularly fast-food restaurants. Restaurants often add sugar and fat to their meals because we, the consumer, like them that way.

Take snacks with you if you are trapped in a fast-food restaurant. Your urge to munch will be nearly irresistible in this setting. Many diet programs offer a variety of take along snacks. These are real life savers. He who lives by fast food, dies (or gets fat) by fast food. Write this on a sticky note and paste it on the dash of your car.

I was able to eat in restaurants without major problems. I decided what I would order before I arrived, and I stuck to my decision. I usually ordered a salad. Many dieters complain that restaurants don't have any low carb items. That's not true for many restaurants, including fast-food restaurants, in my experience. What these folks are really saying is that they don't want to eat what's on their diet. If you find yourself making this complaint, it means that you aren't psychologically prepared to eat out.

Joyner and colleagues also rather cavalierly recommend that you eat only with people who are on your diet. For all practical purposes that translates into no family or group meals. That might work if you live alone. But, most folks don't.

Let's try to make reasonable sense of this recommendation. If you have a supportive family or you are a great persuader, everyone in the household goes on your low carbohydrate diet—a health win for everyone. If your family doesn't eat what you do, you will face some tough choices. You'll have to consider mealtime. Do you lay down martial law and order everyone to eat what you do? Do you eat your meals together or separately? Do you want to miss the time with your husband or kids if you do eat separately? Do you cook foods you can't eat? We don't believe you can cook without tasting or sampling. Sampling leads to cravings. What are you going to feed your kids? Are they old enough to fend for themselves? If your kids are younger, why not get them off to a healthy start? Do them a favor and break their addictions along with yours. What do you do when your daughter wants fast food? My counselor, Barb, doesn't feed her grandchildren junk food when they visit. They eat what she eats. One of them asked her, "Are we going to have normal food?" You'll have to decide how to handle the kids (both adults and children) in your life.

Don't eat anything from a box, a package, or a can. This includes foods prepared for you in take-out wrappers or boxes. It also includes manufactured sauces and spreads (even the so-called healthy ones). Use frozen foods carefully. Many frozen foods are enhanced with sugar and fat. If you use these, read the labels to rule out unwanted additives. It took me 15 minutes to find a package of frozen peas without additives! They were hidden in a forgotten corner of the freezer section. If you do follow this rule, you won't be exposed to the added sugars and unhealthy fats in these products. It is the sugars loaded on top of fats that feed your addiction.

Become a fringe shopper. Shop only the outer edges of the supermarket. Stay away from the inner aisles where highly processed foods hang out. Think of the bakery section as a battlefield filled with land mines. Be a fringe shopper for at least two months. You can then begin to use a few of these products.

Don't eat fresh fruits for at least two weeks. The fructose in fruit is less addictive than processed sugar, but it still feeds an addiction. After eight months, I still cannot eat fruits at will. When I do, I get sugar cravings. I can eat six or seven strawberries and a small bowl of green grapes. If I eat more, the cravings and weight gain begin. Test your limits. Some of you may be less vulnerable to fructose than I am.

Interference Tasks to Block Cravings

Because cravings last only seconds to minutes before they weaken, there are ways to block them by engaging in competing activities (Skorka-Brown et al., 2015). Because cravings place demands on working memory capacity, they can be interrupted by other tasks using the same working memory channel. To understand working memory, try to repeat a 10-digit number while dialing a friend. You can't do it. You must devote all your working memory to the number you're rehearsing or the one you're dialing. The mental tug you feel when trying to do two similar tasks at once is your working memory blowing a fuse. Using interference tasks has been shown to shorten cigarette, food, and coffee cravings (Skorka-Brown et al., 2015).

Interference tasks suppress a craving by pushing it out of working memory. Not all activities are equal when it comes to blocking out cravings. Visual, olfactory, and taste sensations paired with mental activities are the most powerful. Reciting the alphabet backwards or counting backwards, for example, won't crowd out a craving. Auditory tasks like listening to music or humming a tune don't drown out cravings. Pinching yourself won't stop a craving. Imagery, particularly visuospatial imagery, is the most effective interference task. Visual imagery processing makes strong demands on the limited capacity of working memory. Tasks that involve olfactory processing can also be effective.

Binge eaters listen up! If you, like me, eat every potato chip in the package or every candy in the bag, you must have an interference technique which will interrupt your cravings. If you don't have a plan, you are extremely vulnerable to relapse.

These interference tasks won't put an end to your cravings. They will simply stop a specific craving. The potency of these tasks doesn't seem to diminish over time. The several interference tasks you may consider are presented in order of increasing effectiveness (from least to most). Pick the task which best fits your style. If it doesn't work, choose another.

Eat a Substitute Food

You can eat a substitute food when you have a craving. This is a good quick fix. I eat a dill pickle (5 calories and no carbs). The vinegary taste ends my craving. I also like a small piece of cheese, a few walnuts, or a teaspoon of almond butter. This intervention works when you have access to a refrigerator. I don't carry pickles with me when I leave home. Some dieters carry a bottle of water with a tablespoon of vinegar per eight ounces. Other dieters suggest drinking protein powder mixed with water every three to four hours. Finding a protein source without sugar, artificial sweeteners, or caffeine is tricky. We recommend Now Sports Whey Protein Isolate, natural and unflavored. It has 25 grams of protein in a scoop. I find that ½ scoop is enough. Low carbohydrate weight loss programs often sell proprietary protein drinks. Often these are flavored and have sugar substitutes.

Keep a Cravings Diary

There are cellphone applications which help you track your cravings. We've yet to find an app we can recommend. Many of the apps aren't based on science and aren't compatible with a low carbohydrate diet. Stopping and entering data about the length and character of the craving (visual, taste, smell) into a program can be helpful. You can use a notebook or pocket calendar instead. Jot down this information: Sensory property of craving (visual, smell, taste), food craved, and what action you took. This interference task is not powerful, and it does require consistency and the right environment. You must be able to take a moment to write the craving information down.

Urge Surfing

Urge surfing is a technique which was introduced in substance addiction treatment. Urge surfing is a fun way of saying "go with your craving, don't fight it." You allow the craving to come to you, you observe it as it moves, and you go with it in the manner of a surfer following the crest of a wave, hence, the name urge surfing. In other words, think of the craving as a wave you're riding, not an enemy. Urge surfing is a mindfulness technique. There is a large literature on the use of mindfulness techniques to control alcohol and drug cravings. This technique works because it diminishes the emotional power of a craving.

Fighting a craving means you are thinking about it. You are giving the craving power, a space in your mind. Mindfulness suggests that you come to peace with your cravings and stop battling them. The upside of urge surfing is its availability. You can urge surf anywhere and at any time. The downside is the learning curve. Mindfulness is a mental control technique, and you must practice it. The learning curve is not long, but it will take a week or two to get reliable benefits from urge surfing. Mindfulness is trendy at this writing. You can find many references on the Internet or in your local library. Trainers are also available.

Imagining a Favorite Activity

Imagining a favorite activity when cravings strike can reduce their intensity making the cravings pass by more quickly. People who had strong cravings for specific foods or drinks, most often coffee or chocolate, were asked to imagine a favorite activity whenever they had a craving. Imagining worked better than overlearned tasks like reciting the alphabet backwards, humming, or counting (Skorka-Brown et al., 2015). The image must engage your mind.

To use this technique, first develop a list of things to imagine. You can't just pull one out of thin air when cravings happen. The topics can be favorite things, places, events, or people. I like to remember what the moon looked like one romantic night by a lake. It's best that the images don't involve food. Good examples are visiting a zoo and watching the lions sun themselves, watching a sunset across the ocean, or reaching the top of a mountain and looking at the valley below. The list of possibilities is endless. Once you have your list, carry it with you. When the next craving happens, and it will, imagine the item for approximately three minutes. Three minutes seems to be the bare minimum time to block a craving.

You may think you're not good at creating mental pictures. The quality or vividness of your visual images is not important (McClelland, Kemps, & Tiggemann, 2006). It's trying to imagine a picture that's important.

Reward Yourself

This is an old behavioral technique which has stood the test of time. The technique is best explained by example. Years ago, I was asked to lead a stop-smoking group by the American Cancer Society. I didn't want to because I was smoking 10 cigarettes per day at the time. After I thought about leading the stop-smoking group, I decided it was an opportunity to end my nicotine addiction.

One of the techniques used in the program was the following: Each time you crave a cigarette and don't respond, reward yourself. Each time you crave a cigarette and smoke, do something non-rewarding. It's best if the reward is tangible and easily seen. The reward can be as simple as a gold star on a calendar and a red devil sticker for each lapse. Each client in the smoking group chose their own reward. I decided to save the money I was spending on cigarettes for a trip to Mexico. For each craving I passed, I put $1.00 in a jar. For each craving I couldn't control, I bought a pack of cigarettes, took one cigarette from the pack, smoked it, and threw the package of cigarettes in the trash. When I got home, I put $5.00 in a jar to be donated to the American Cancer Foundation.

I didn't find any recent research using this approach with carbohydrate addiction; however, it was combined with video game playing by Hsu and colleagues (2014) to good advantage.

Do Eye-hand or Movement Activities

Do something with both hands. I like needlework and beading. You can't eat when doing needlepoint; however, these activities aren't always convenient. We found no research on other motor activities such as exercise or vacuuming. You can test them out.

Sniff a Non-food Scent

There's good research support for sniffing a non–food odorant such as eucalyptus, musk, or jasmine to interrupt a craving. As odd as it may seem, smelling something other than food is one of the most powerful ways to derail a carbohydrate craving.

There are many essential oils available. Don't select a food odor such as lemon, orange, cinnamon, etc. You could also carry a small jar of Mentholatum or Vicks rub. We suspect that stronger scents such as cedar or eucalyptus will work better, but we can't prove this. Keep the selected scent with you. Since it takes at least three minutes for an intervention to have any effect, you may have to sniff more than once.

Play Video Games

If you pair sound with a visual experience, cravings can be passed by without damage to your resolution. An early study looked at the ability of sound to interfere with cravings. In one paradigm, noise and a visual display (called dynamic visual noise) were used as an interference task with individuals who were addicted to cigarettes and food. We don't have visual noise generators at our disposal, so investigators turned to video games. These games have a visual display and make a variety of sounds. Hsu and colleagues chose *Tetris* because it is available to most of us, and many versions can be downloaded at no cost (Hsu et al., 2014).

Tetris involves manipulating colored shapes such as squares to form rows which would extend the game. The game requires mental rotation and movement. When the participants in the study (college students) had a craving, they filled out a questionnaire about the craving and then played *Tetris* for three minutes. One of the questions was whether they had indulged the craving. They then went back to their regular college activities. Other students filled out the questionnaire, but they didn't play *Tetris*. The researchers found that playing *Tetris* for three minutes decreased craving strength for nicotine, alcohol, caffeine, and food by 80%. Only one craving in five was acted upon.

Smile

This is our personal favorite. Maybe smiling won't help you avoid cravings as well as playing *Tetris*, but it might boost the strength of the other interference tasks. Smiling works by breaking the link between eating craved foods and our negative emotions (Schmidt & Martin, 2017). Let's face it. Cravings are depressing!

One of the most fascinating research findings in the last few years was the link between the way our emotions are felt and the way they are expressed. If we are angry, for example, we frown. We show this on our faces by changing the activity of the corrugator muscles of our face. If we are happy, we smile. We modulate the zygomatic muscles of our face. The nuances of our emotions and how they are shown on our faces has been categorized. In our brains, the feelings of sadness or happiness produce distinct brain activities. Now comes the interesting part. If you ask an accomplished actor to use his facial muscles to mimic basic emotions, the brain activities are identical to the "real" emotions.

How does this work with cravings? The theory suggests that our facial expressions can produce emotions as well as being the result of our emotions. Thus, smiling while experiencing a craving can change the emotions or the negativity of the craving. In the study, subjects were asked to smile or frown when they had food cravings caused by seeing highly desired foods. The researchers found that smiling decreased cravings.

Smiling is particularly important for those of us who eat to treat negative feelings. If you eat a box of chocolate after a difficult talk with your boss, you are an emotional eater. This technique might work well for you. Here's an example of how to use this technique. Instead of eating that chocolate, think of the silliest thing your boss ever did, think about your favorite scene in a funny movie, tell a joke to a co-worker, or think about your child's sweetest gift to you, etc. Even if this technique isn't strong enough to beat your cravings, it always helps to smile more.

Exercise

Come up with a cravings management plan. You'll need to look at shopping, cooking, meal sharing, and cravings interference. Spending a little time here may just mean the difference between successful weight management or more of the same.

CHAPTER 14

We may find in the long run that tinned food is a deadlier weapon than the machine gun. — George Orwell

Overcoming Our Programming

Many of us enjoy talking about food. I know I do. Admit it. You're with friends here. If you're a carbohydrate addict, you do too. We talk about food because we're obsessed. Food is uppermost in our minds. Somewhere in our heads, either at the back or front of our consciousness, we're thinking about food—when we will eat, where we will eat, and what we will eat. This may come as a shock, but many people aren't obsessed with food. These strange creatures don't give a hang about food. What they eat, or whether they eat at all, is a matter of no consequence. I married one of these odd people. It will come as no surprise that he isn't a carbohydrate addict. He comes from a family whose lives don't revolve around food. As you might expect, no one in his family struggles with his or her weight.

So what's the point, you may be asking yourself. The point is simple and generally overlooked in diet books. We overeat because of the way we think about food. To overcome a carbohydrate addiction, we must change the way we think. Consider the alcoholic again. An alcoholic must revamp the role alcohol plays in his or her life—no more martinis before dinner to unwind, no champagne on New Year's Eve, no more drinks to celebrate a promotion, no alcohol to soothe wounded feelings, etc. Putting it simply, to lose weight, changing the types of foods you eat isn't enough. You must change the way you think about food. You must change what food means to you. Unfortunately, we know very little about how to go about this. We'll share what we do know. You'll forgive us if we struggle and stumble as we write this chapter because we're entering relatively uncharted territory.

* * * *

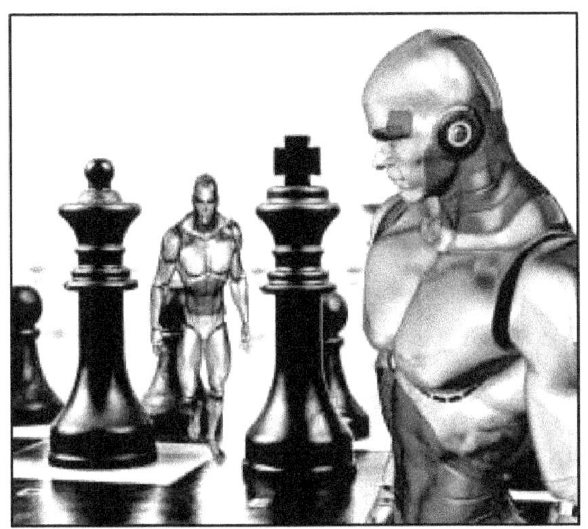

One way to understand food programming is to imagine you're a robot with a computer for a brain. When your creator started tinkering, you were a blank slate. You had no preferences, no rules. However, your creators (or parents) immediately started programming you to behave in certain ways. Because you are not the creator, you must do what the creators say, or eat what your creators eat and will let you eat. This is how our food programming begins.

Image by <a href="https://pixabay.com/users/Owensart-2185191/

Other little robots, programmed by different creators, are learning different rules. For some of us, food is immensely pleasurable. For others, food is far down their list of sensory experiences. When our food programming is completed, we think of ourselves as in charge of our brains and our programming. The bad news is we're not in charge. We never have been, and we never will be. What we can do is make ourselves aware of our programming and move it step by step onto healthier ground. Always remember, it took a lifetime to program your personal robot brain.

In the previous chapter, we talked about techniques for interrupting cravings. Stopping cravings is the essential first step in reprogramming the way we eat. Cravings, those automatic, powerful food commands, are the most obvious primary manifestation of our food programming. Stopping cravings must happen before any other changes in our programming can begin. We must tell our robot brain we are in charge, and it can keep nagging forever. "Go ahead robot brain, talk. I won't listen."

The next step is more challenging. We've stopped the cravings, but how do we change less automatic thought processes, particularly those tied to our emotions? A typical scenario goes like this. You're driving to work. You've had breakfast and sent your kids to school. Thoughts of all kinds dash about in your brain. Did you remember to turn on the slow cooker? What's wrong with the driver ahead of you? Doesn't he know how to use a turn signal? You wonder if you sent your son back to school too soon after his bout with a cold. Then, you think of the chicken soup your mother always made when you were sick. You feel guilty. You're lazy because you were too tired to make soup for your son. You really are a terrible parent. If your son gets pneumonia, it'll be your fault. You see a doughnut store. You stop at that store and you buy a wonderful doughnut stuffed with raspberry jelly. The relief is immediate, but brief. You get back in your car thinking you are weak and worthless. And so the cycle goes on and on and on.

There are two basic psychotherapeutic approaches which have been used to change the way we think and the way we behave. The first is change from the inside to the outside. We change our thoughts, and our altered way of thinking brings about different actions. A good example of this is cognitive therapy. You talk to your therapist about your frustration with your wife because she insists you put the toilet seat down, but she never returns the favor. The therapist suggests that you discuss the problem with your spouse and tell her how angry this makes you. You want her to understand, so she'll change what she does.

The other method is to change from the outside to the inside. We don't worry about what's going on in our noodles. We just change our environment and our relationship to it, and our thoughts will follow. Using the same example, our therapist suggests that you put a sign on one of the bathroom doors stating that this bathroom is for gents only. You've changed your environment. Problem solved.

Much ink has been spilt by psychologists debating just this dichotomy. Is it better to focus on what we think (cognitive therapy) or to focus on what we do and not worry so much about what we think (behavior therapy)? In other words, does behavior follow thoughts or do thoughts follow behavior? We'll talk about ways to change our programming using both approaches. You'll note that some of these techniques were also used to stop cravings.

Working from the Inside Out

There are fewer cognitive approaches to changing our food programming, but we can draw from therapy approaches to other common problems. One important approach is to make your implicit thought processes explicit. We get used to letting our robot brains rattle on and on about all kinds of things including what foods we're going to eat. How do we change this?

Tell Your Story

Your story is unique, and it's important. You can't know how to go about changing unless you know what you want to change. The first thing any therapist worth his pay does is take your history. Knowing our history paves our way to our futures. Patients were often puzzled when I asked so many questions about their siblings, children, job, finances, etc. All they wanted to know was how to get their spouse to do things their way. You've probably never really thought about your food history. It's unlikely that you've ever shared your food story. If you like to write, you can jot down your history beginning with your first food memory. Don't stop there, go through your food memories year by year. Which food memories stand out in grade school, middle school, or high school? Telling your story is a good first step at making the implicit explicit.

Many of us don't like to write. You can start with this. Every time you think of a food you dislike write it down in a simple notebook. You can also do this for foods you like. Later when you have a moment, think about the strong feeling of liking or disliking. Where and when did it begin. Was there a trauma linked to this dislike? If you find yourself with many dislikes, you probably have an eating disorder. Losing weight will be more problematic if you have an eating disorder beyond overeating. If this fits you, think about seeing a therapist to help you unravel your food related thoughts and feelings. Since you're a carbohydrate addict, one thing is certain. You adore every sugar and starch ever invented, but you may have strong dislikes for other foods.

Then there are those odd people—the ones who don't care much about food. They tend to have short lists of foods they don't like. The reason is simple. They don't have many strong preferences. Food is food. One of the beautiful things about my husband's parents was their flexibility. You could take them to any restaurant, and they ate what was put in front of them with no complaints. Conversely, I could bust my tail preparing an exotic meal, and they wouldn't notice. These odd people don't need cookbooks. If you ask them to tell you what they had for lunch, they might not remember. Food doesn't register in their odd little heads.

Food Memories Count

We addicts tend to have strong food memories. When I drive by a restaurant, memories fill my brain. I remember what I ordered and whether I liked it or not. I even remember events before and after the meal. My odd husband, on the other hand, sometimes isn't sure if he ate at the restaurant. He often doesn't remember what he ate (or care much either). He doesn't use food to mark events. I do.

At first blush, food memories might not strike you as an important part of addiction, but they are. As it turns out, we often choose foods based not on what they taste like but what we remember about them (Hoogeveen et al., 2016). We rely upon previous experience more than actual taste when we select foods. We certainly don't choose foods because of their health properties. Consider this example. For years, I wouldn't eat eggs for breakfast. Eggs, particularly fried eggs, made me nauseous. Why? I experienced a traumatic separation from my mother when I was five years old. During her absence, my father fixed my meals. What did he cook? You guessed it, fried eggs morning, noon, and night. It took many years before I could enjoy fried eggs for breakfast.

Your memories of your favorite carbohydrates have tremendous power. Does the chocolate turtle taste heavenly or are you remembering feeling better in the past after you ate chocolate? One way to change the way you think is to find ways to celebrate that don't involve food. Make a list of things you can do to celebrate. For example, go to a movie (no stops at the concession stand), take a walk, buy flowers, go on a drive, play cards, etc. Have these ready when you have a food celebration urge.

Expectations Pave the Way

Next look at your expectations. Food tastes the way we expect it to taste. Taste is not absolute. Our sense of taste is not like a thermometer. It doesn't give exact readings. One experiment illustrates the point. Young men thought they were being given two kinds of baloney, regular or reduced fat. Because they expected the fattier baloney to taste better, they rated a baloney sample labeled as having a higher fat content as tasting better than samples marked low fat. In truth, the baloney samples had the same amount of fat. It was the men's expectation of taste which made the baloney taste better (Myers, 2015). If you don't like spicy food and a friend suggests lunch at a Thai restaurant, you are likely to expect that the food will be spicier than you like. The simple knowledge that you're in a Thai restaurant will prime your expectation. No matter how spicy the food is, it will be experienced as too spicy and rejected.

Beware of your food expectations. They aren't trustworthy. Improve your awareness of your expectations and try to go against them. Rather than declining an invitation to go to a Thai restaurant with a friend, accept the invitation and search through the menu until you find something you can eat. There's something on every menu you can eat. We promise you. Ask the server for samples of foods you haven't tried. Taste them with an open mind. Don't stop with one taste. Taste three or four times to allow your expectations to shift. You might be surprised by the result. Similarly, become aware of your expectation that all sweets taste good. Many don't if you take a moment and really taste them. Some of them are stale, and many are adulterated with all manner of chemicals and additives.

Our expectations also influence the amount we eat or drink. If we're told that a beverage is unsweetened, we will drink more than if it's labeled as containing sugar. We'll taste sweetness based on our expectation, not the amount of sugar which the drink contains. We don't like the taste of unsweetened beverages, for example, because the first sip doesn't match our expectation. If we don't know the sugar content, we can be fooled just like with baloney samples. I am reminded of a trick we used to play. In my college, we were divided into Pepsi or Coke drinkers. We had strong preferences for one or the other. We swore that we could tell them apart. When we gave a strong believer a taste challenge, he or she often couldn't tell Pepsi from Coke. It is the label on the bottle that tells us what the taste will be. Our addicted brains fill in the sensory details.

Too Much Variety

Although we think of taste as stable—the first bite of a cookie is the same as the last—taste sensations change with each bite we take and each time the food is eaten. This is due to two opposing neural processes, sensitization and habituation (Myers, 2015). When we first see or anticipate a food we like, the body prepares to eat by starting digestive processes. This is sensitization. The brain, amped up by our expectations, enhances the flavor of that first bite.

Habituation happens when you continue to eat the same food. The pleasure of each bite is less than the one before. Habituation helps regulate how much we eat.

Habituation and sensitization have been studied with animals. If a hungry rat or mouse is placed in a maze with a reward at the end, it will run faster and work harder to get to that reward. With time, the animal habituates. Now, the still hungry animal runs slower and will do less work to get to the reward. Eventually, the animal goes to sleep in the maze! You might argue that the animal is simply full. All you must do is change the reward, and the sleepy animal will run and work as before.

To know the truth of this for us, consider this situation. You sit down to eat a piece of pie. The first bite takes you straight to heaven. The second bite is good but not ecstasy producing. By the sixth bite, you may be eating mechanically. You might be watching the news scarcely noticing the pie. Loss of pleasure or habituation also happens across meals with the same food. Suppose you made an enormous stew. The first night it tastes wonderful. By the end of a week, you can't stand the thought of it, so you throw it away.

We can use habituation to our benefit in weight loss by eating the same meals each day. It may be tiresome, but you'll eat less without even trying due to our friend habituation. If we go back and look at the lives of those odd people who don't care about food, they often don't vary their menus. They're happy eating the same breakfast, lunch, and dinner day after day. These folks are examples of habituation in its most extreme form.

I was brought up in a household by a mother who loved to cook. Every night, she prepared something different. When I oversaw meal planning as an adult, I carried my mother's pattern forward. As a newlywed, I felt it was my obligation to cook something different each day. I have only recently understood how I had become obsessed with food and why I had struggled to control my weight. I was doing everything wrong. I was trying to challenge my taste buds with new and different meals. I thought this made me a good cook and a good homemaker. What I was actually doing was focusing too much of my energy on food. I was preventing the normal process of habituation from helping me control the amount of food I ate. I was making me and everyone around me gain weight.

Don't take all the blame. Our culture is setting us up to want more and different kinds of food. There was a time when Chinese, Italian, and Mexican restaurants were considered exotic. Most cafes served the same basic meals. Now, every major city has all manner of cuisine. Some of it is so exotic that I'm not sure what it is, e.g., Asian fusion. This variety is not bad in and of itself. Variety is pleasing, but too much variety increases the likelihood we will gain weight. Variety sensitizes the taste buds. Food manufacturers know we'll eat a larger amount if the food is highly-flavored. To augment food tastes, they've gone to flavor boosters. If we eat more, we buy more. That solves their problem, but it makes us fat.

Now, I don't mark my success by the complexity and diversity of my meals. The slow cooker is my new best friend. I make large amounts of everything. I eat the same meals for days. I let my friend habituation help me. Are you hooked on novelty?

Working from the Outside In

Most diet books focus on these approaches. Authors tell us to get all carbohydrate loaded foods out of the house. They tell us to eat slowly and taste what we eat. Why? These methods work.

Let me give you an example from my life of how changing your actions can change your thinking. Because I am obsessed with food, I always plan the holiday meals well in advance. I look up recipes in my cookbook trying to find the perfect combination of foods. I make lists to be sure that I have enough ingredients in the refrigerator. I think about the layout of the Christmas table before I go to sleep. By Christmas day, I'm ready. My mother did the same thing. She started asking what we wanted for Christmas dinner shortly after Thanksgiving. She made sure we would be there to eat her dinner about the same time. Missing her Christmas dinner would have wounded her to her core. This year to my surprise, I forgot about Christmas dinner. I realized with a start that I hadn't done one single thing to prepare for Christmas dinner, and Christmas was only five days away. Somehow during the year of cutting back on carbohydrates, I'd changed. My way of thinking about food had followed.

In the next section, we'll look at a few actions you can take to improve your control of your addiction.

Try Spices

If your spice shelf consists of a few outdated jars of cinnamon, cloves, and nutmeg, it's time to expand your horizons. Use spices to change your idea of how good sugary foods taste. Spices can get our addicted taste buds to accept lower sugar and lower fat versions of foods. Best of all, spices don't add calories or sugar. They're nature's gifts. In one study, researchers added spices to three types of foods—a non-sugar item to which sugar is often added (tea), an item with a small amount of built in sugar to which sugar is often added (oatmeal with dried apples), and a food with tons of sugar (apple crisp with apples plus additional recipe sugar) (Peters, Marker, Pan, Breen, & Hill, 2018). Spices were added to increase the flavor profile of some, but not all, mixtures, and people were asked how well they liked the taste. When spices were added to apple crisp, for example, sugar levels could be reduced by 37% and the degree of liking or enjoyment stayed the same.

Giving up sugar is best, but if you need a slower approach, retune your taste buds by gradually cutting back the amount of sugar you use. After bariatric surgery, patients reported that sweet foods were less pleasing (Nance, Eagon, Klein, & Pepino, 2017). I also experienced this. As a life-long Coca Cola addict, I now find the taste too sugary, to the point of tasting unpleasant. What happened? My taste buds had adapted and developed a new normal. An Asian woman of my acquaintance pointed out that Asian desserts don't contain as much sugar. She can't tolerate an American made cheesecake. I tried the Asian bakery she recommended. She was right. Their cheesecake was not as sweet. They've tuned their taste buds to expect less sugar.

Most recipes can be made with less sugar. Although its wiser to abandon sugar all together, that isn't realistic for all of us. If you eat desserts, make them yourself so you can control the sugar in them. Then reduce the amount of sugar the recipe recommends.

Learn to Like Vegetables

Carbohydrate addicts who don't eat vegetables face a more challenging recovery. Let's get real here. Vegetables are a central food group when you go on a low carbohydrate diet. Our liking for healthy foods like vegetables can be changed. It can be conditioned. An example of negative conditioning (decreasing our liking of a food) is the aversive conditioning I described when I ate a bad clam. One bite of one clam was enough to make me avoid clams and anything resembling a clam. To induce negative conditioning for a food one craves, add something disliked. This reduces the likelihood that we'll eat the food again.

We can positively condition our liking of less preferred foods such as cauliflower or kale by using a process called flavor-flavor conditioning. When a neutral, novel, or disliked flavor is consumed with another taste or flavor that is pleasant, our appreciation of the neutral, novel, or disliked flavor is improved. For example, if you give a child a new flavor, let's say green beans, which they haven't experienced, they're more likely to enjoy it if it is mixed with a little sugar or extra butter. When the child tastes beans again, he or she will like the taste. In another example, adults learn to enjoy herbal teas by tasting them first with sugar.

The best positive flavors to use are fatty or sugary substances. For example, someone who dislikes kale might like it in a salad with bacon dressing. The positive effects of pairings are weaker than aversive conditioning and often take several trials.

Myers (2015) recommended that the amount of a positive flavor added to a less liked food be decreased gradually. Let's take coffee as an example. If someone who doesn't like coffee adds milk and sugar, the coffee is more palatable. Over time, we decrease the amount of sugar and milk. We have learned to like coffee at a much higher concentration. Myer described a study in a college dormitory where students didn't eat some of the vegetables. If the vegetables were flavored with sauces and spices, the students reported a greater liking for the vegetable. More importantly, the students ate more vegetables.

In several experiments with children, the young participants changed their rankings of new foods faster if they had experienced the flavor paired with added calories.

If you struggle to eat your veggies, add butter, fruits, or simple fat-based sauces. You can add a little applesauce to your spinach. We don't recommend buying the packaged versions of vegetables because you cannot control the amounts of sugar and fat when you use this approach. You do need to gradually decrease the additives until you are able to eat it as nature intended.

Context Counts

Be aware of where you eat and with whom. The social effect of the context in which foods are presented is extremely important in the formation of our eating preferences. We're taught that making mealtime special is a good idea. Unfortunately, we've taken this idea much too seriously. It's a good idea to stop and enjoy what we eat but making meals special also supports addiction when taken to extremes. Look at Thanksgiving for example. This holiday has grown into an occasion to gorge and eat all manner of carbohydrates.

Context can be a useful tool. For example, young children's eating habits can be molded using context. When children are told that a previously neutral or unknown food is a reward, they often like it. If children are given a neutral treat and they are given positive attention, they often like the treat. If children are given a neutral food at snack time without attention or suggestion that it's a reward, they are less likely to enjoy it (Hoogeveen et al., 2016; Myers, 2015).

I became acutely aware of context the first week of my low carbohydrate diet. My menu called for four ounces of cooked (8 ounces raw) vegetables at each meal including breakfast. Do you know how many bites of salad it takes to make up eight ounces? Do you eat salad or broccoli for breakfast? Now, a little green pepper and tomatoes in an omelette is okay, but a salad? We learn to eat certain foods at certain times. Breakfast is the context in which we eat eggs or cereal. We eat salads with dinner or lunch, right? The context in which foods are usually consumed becomes our normal, our standard.

The effect of context is significant. If we are given foods we don't expect at a meal, we'll eat less. If we're in a context in which we normally eat the food, we'll eat more. What's more, we feel satisfied when we eat the foods we expect at our normal times. Play with the context in which you eat food groups. Eat breakfast foods for dinner, dinner foods for breakfast, and breakfast foods for lunch, etc. Change the order in which you eat your foods. Challenge your habits.

Context also misleads us. If we believe that we've eaten something healthy, we feel more satisfied afterward. Unfortunately, this leads us to rely on the information on packages. If a cereal box shows us a decathlon athlete on the front and tells us that the cereal inside is heart healthy, we believe this although most of these products are loaded with refined carbohydrates and are not in the least heart healthy. I ate cereal for breakfast for years. I made it taste a little less like cardboard by adding sugar and raisins. After searching every cereal product on the planet, we found only one which was acceptable given my new appreciation of my carbohydrate addiction. Fiber One. That's a very sad commentary when you think of all the pricey cereals labeled organic, heart healthy, etc.

Our choice of dining companions also affects our food preferences and consumption. We eat more in the presence of others (Ertmans, Baeyens, & Bergh, 2002). One consistently reported fact is that married couples weigh more than single individuals. Why? Couples tend to eat together. Going to any shared meal should be viewed as entering a dangerous carbohydrate jungle. Be very aware of what you eat in any social situation. It's best to plan what you're going to eat before you go to a shared meal. Decide what you will eat and stick to your plan.

For the Artificial Sweetener Addict

Addiction to artificially sweetened beverages is difficult to beat. We can pass along one good tip. Many artificial sweeteners have a metallic taste when served at room temperature. Make a pact to drink these drinks only at room temperature. You'll discover what the chemicals really taste like. The developers of these sweeteners invested hundreds of thousands of dollars to create a sweetener that would taste good when cold. Undercut their efforts to get this nasty stuff into your body!

Exercise

Look at the programming problems related to eating. Which do you have? What can you do to change your programming? Make a list of those you might want to change.

OVERVIEW OF PROGRAMMING ISSUES

- Have you thought about your eating history? You might have traumatic memories or other destructive conditioning.
- Do you dislike vegetables? Learn to eat more vegetables.
- Is it hard for you to avoid eating with others, situations which lead to overeating, or eating the wrong foods? Ask your counselor and friends for suggestions.
- Do you have a narrow range of foods you like or, conversely, are you hooked on novelty when it comes to food? Think about ways to change.
- Are you conditioned to eat certain foods at certain times? Fiddle with foods and times you eat them (i.e., breakfast foods at dinner).
- Are you an emotional eater? Pay attention to your emotional state. Find other ways to soothe yourself (hot shower, call a good friend, take a walk with your dog).
- Do many situations evoke strong feelings and memories linked to carbohydrate binges? Notice these situations and find ways to avoid them as much as possible.

CHAPTER 15

Guilt is a rope that wears thin. —Ayn Rand

Nobody Loves a Fat Man

Why are we obsessed with skinny? Why are we pursuing ridiculously teeny tiny bodies when we should be obsessed with health? The medical profession is also obsessed with weight rather than health. The truth is thin people can have poor health, and many overweight people enjoy long lives and good health. Our obsessive over-emphasis on skinny is the root cause of the O-word stigma. A stigma is a mark of disgrace. Bearing a stigma means its owner should be ashamed. Our stigmatization of overweight persons is damaging, and we must stop doing it. Most importantly, we must stop stigmatizing ourselves because feeling ashamed of ourselves and our bodies increases the likelihood that we'll remain overweight and maybe even pile on a few more pounds.

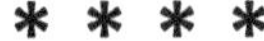

Don't Be Defeated

Don't be ashamed of your weight. What you've gained, you can lose. One of the first things to change is how you describe yourself. I used to be corpulent—the word has a nice ring to it. I'm not obese. Obesity is an ugly word. Let's not use the "O" word when referring to ourselves. Leave this word to the scientists and medical professionals. I'd rather be called fat. The O-word is derived from the Latin word "obesus" which has two meanings. The first meaning is becoming plump through eating, but the second meaning is being coarse or vulgar (Barnett, 2005). The O-word first appeared in a medical context in a book titled *Via Recta* by Thomas Venner (1620). Venner believed obesity was an occupational hazard of the civilized class, and he believed their "physique" could be restored by following the concepts of Hippocrates (balanced diet, sleep, etc.). As time passed, the word obesity picked up additional baggage. The negative reference suggesting that a high BMI was vulgar was replaced by moral indictments. The overweight individual was guilty of a crime against himself, and he must take personal responsibility. Thus, to be guilty of the O-word, you are coarse, vulgar, fat, morally weak, and irresponsible.

Stigmatization of individuals with high BMI is not new. Banting wrote "A Letter on Corpulence Addressed to The Public" in 1863. In the 18th and 19th centuries, writers preferred the term "corpulence" or "excessively fat". Banning wrote:

"Obesity seems to me very little understood or properly appreciated by the faculty and the public generally or the former would long ere this have hit upon the cause for so lamentable a disease, and applied effective remedies, whilst the latter would have spared their injudicious indulgence in remarks and sneers, frequently painful in society, and which, even on the stronger mind, have an unhappy tendency; but I sincerely trust this humble effort at exposition may lead to a more perfect ventilation of the subject and a better feeling for the afflicted."

Banting is credited with publishing the first diet program, and his pamphlet describes the many cures he tried and the number of experts he consulted before he found a diet that worked for him. He tried rowing, sea air bathing, gallons of physic and liquor potasse, horseback riding, the waters at Leamington, and Turkish baths. He eventually found an expert who educated him on sugar and starch. He lost 46 pounds on this diet, and he shared his diet and his experiences in the pamphlet. He concluded:

"For the sake of argument and illustration, I will presume that certain articles of ordinary diet, however beneficial in youth, are prejudicial in advanced life, like beans to a horse, whose common ordinary food is hay and corn. It may be useful food occasionally under peculiar circumstances, but detrimental as a constancy. I will, therefore, adopt the analogy, and call such food human

beans. The items from which I was advised to abstain as much as possible were bread, butter, milk, sugar, beer and potatoes, which had been the main (and I thought innocent) elements of my existence ..."

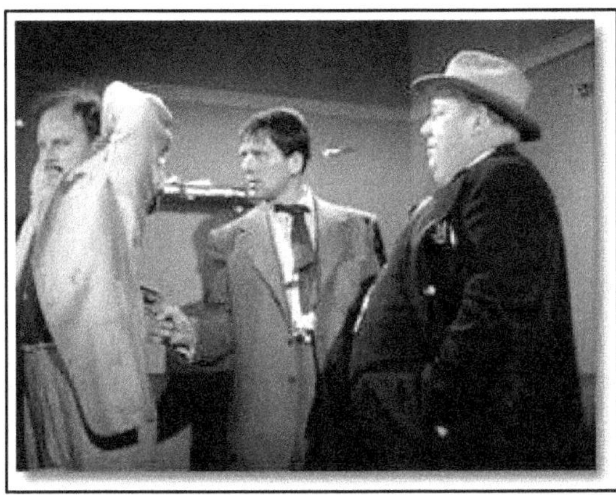

Did you see the 1952 movie, *Narrow Margin?* The super-sized railroad detective shown to the right of the photograph had a girth large enough to fill the narrow train corridors. At one point when the corridor is crowded with irritated passengers trying to move past him, he says with a chuckle, "Nobody loves a fat man." His statement summarizes the stigma associated with being overweight in a skinny-crazed world. A traveler wrote a wonderful letter about being the fat lady on an airplane flight. https://medium.com/s/story/a-letter-from-the-fat-person-on-your-flight-b0ceb1407c61 Check out *Dietland* on AMC. Also read *The Elephant in the Room: One Fat Man's Quest to Get Smaller in Growing America.* Mr. Tomlinson described his experience:

"I flash back to elementary school in Georgia, standing in the aisle on the school bus. The driver hollers at me to find a seat. He can't take us home until everybody sits down. I'm the only one standing. Every time I spot an open space, somebody slides to the edge of the seat and covers it up. Nobody wants the fat boy mashed in next to them. I freeze, helpless."

These folks express the agony of being supersized in a small world much better than we can.

You probably already know this, but some things are worth repeating. First, ridiculing someone because of his or her weight is socially acceptable (Tomlimson, 2019). It shouldn't be, but it is. On an Internet post, a woman described going to a bar with some college friends. A fellow student approached her and asked for her phone number. She watched him walk across the bar and rejoin his friends. The gaggle of males stared, laughed, and pointed. It took her a second to catch on. She'd been a bet, the butt of a joke. The humiliation and shame of this experience never went away.

Jokes are only funny when both people laugh. Write that down. Jokes hurt. A friend from Latin America caught me up short when I made a joke putting someone down. He didn't understand or appreciate American humor. He asked me why we liked to make fun of other people's weaknesses. I had no answer. As I thought about it, I understood that we (meaning United States folks) are expected to accept abuse if the person insults us in a humorous way. We say if our target looks hurt or protests, "I was only joking." We expect the abused person to laugh along with us.

To understand the devastating effect of misplaced humor, consider the following story. A very pretty and intelligent girl is teased by her siblings. They nickname her Baby Huey and call her Fattie. This young girl grows into a woman with poor self-confidence and a weight issue. Was calling her Baby Huey funny? Should we laugh along? No. Jokes are funny only when both parties laugh.

Prejudice about a person's weight is common. Research shows that overweight individuals provoke more feelings of disgust than other marginalized populations—e.g., homeless, mentally ill, etc. (Incollingo Rodriguez, Heldreth, & Tomiyama, 2016). In fact, individuals with high BMIs are at the bottom of the bad joke pyramid. Someone might hesitate before telling a racist or sexist joke, but jokes making fun of fat people and media images of silly fat people are everywhere (Greenberg, Eastin, Hofschire, Lachlan, & Brownell, 2003). In the movie, *The Nutty Professor*, Dr. Klump is told he is a "fat tub of goo." Jay Leno made this lame joke, "Our fat American kids have to write their history notes on potato chips."

What we see on television or in the movies has a major impact on how we think and behave. The process of stigmatizing people because of their weight begins in early childhood. For example, boys who watch a lot of television are more likely to assign negative stereotypes to women with high BMIs (Harrison, 2000).

How does television content produce these negative views? Part of the answer comes from an analysis of children's movies. The 25 top selling children's movies on Amazon and the American Film Institute's top movies were analyzed for weight stigmatization. Overweight characters in these videos have negative traits. They are evil, unattractive, unfriendly, and cruel. Characters with thin bodies have desirable traits like happiness and kindness (Himes & Thompson, 2007).

When we move to content watched by families, the beat goes on. Greenberg looked at 10 fictional television series that were high in the Nielsen ratings (Greenberg et al., 2003). Thinner women are portrayed more positively than larger ones. The higher the BMI of the female character, the more negative comments she receives from the male characters. The high BMI characters hold marginal roles in our society. That is, they are ethnic minorities, older, unmarried, or unemployed. They are passive, and they are often unhelpful. They do not take leadership roles, and they do not date or have sex. Larger characters are more often seen in comedies than in dramas. When shown in dramas, overweight characters are shown eating or as the objects of humor.

There are gender differences in the way the sexes are stereotyped. Male characters are seen in a negative way if they are *either* thin *or* large. Only medium sized men get the job, solve the crime, tell the jokes, or get the girl. Finally, overweight males do not get as many negative comments about their appearance. The audience laughs when an overweight woman is teased, but the audience doesn't laugh when an overweight man is teased about his weight.

Third, stereotyping based on body size is severe. Overweight individuals are stereotyped as lazy, lacking in will power, weak, and unattractive (Brochu & Esses, 2011). Although there are many overweight adults in the United States, there is "no majority privilege associated with being fat." If you're a specific gender or race, you might get to take advantage of positive biases. No such positive bias exists if you're high BMI.

The negative stereotypes linked to your weight go straight to the bone—to your essence, who and what you are. The stereotypes shame us. Shame is a social emotion. It helps control group members. We use it to control our children and teach moral values. We also believe showing shame proves our sincerity. Some scientists have suggested that shame is a fundamental emotional response to threats to our social group (Dickerson, Gruenewald, & Kemeny, 2004). Shame may have evolved to protect us from these threats.

Shame and the Fat Suit

Why talk about shame in a book about carbohydrate addiction? Shame and the associated emotions of anxiety and depression are co-pilots in our carbohydrate addiction. Shame is a key emotion because being overweight in a skinny world elicits a high level of shame (Conradt et al., 2007). Shame sets a vicious physiological cycle involving the hormone cortisol into motion. We'll cover the nuts and bolts of cortisol in the next section.

You don't have to be overweight to experience the shame of being overweight. Individuals with normal body weights who don't like their bodies also feel ashamed. Individuals pretending to have a high BMI also experience shame.

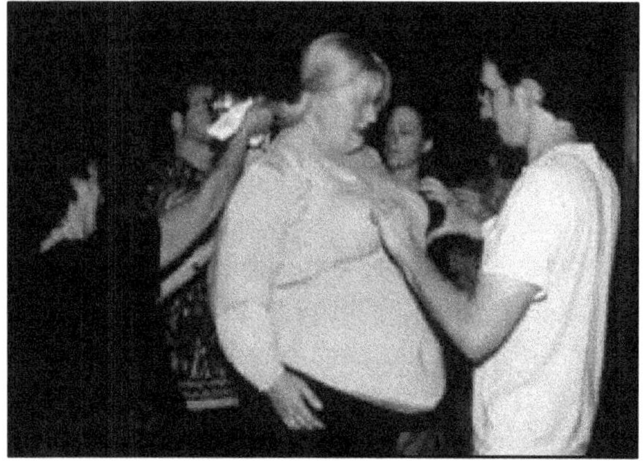

For example, several celebrities have worn fat suit prostheses to experience the effects of obesity. Actors have worn fat suits as part of their roles. Gweneth Paltrow wore a fat suit in the movie, *Shallow Hal.* Early in the shooting, Ms. Paltrow wore the fat suit into her hotel. "The first day I tried (the fat suit) on, I was in the Tribeca Grand Hotel, and I walked across the lobby. It was so sad; it was disturbing. No one would make eye contact with me because I was obese."

Tyra Banks wore a fat suit prosthesis for 15 hours. This was her experience. "The people were staring and laughing in my face—that shocked me the most. As soon as I entered the store—I immediately heard snickers. Immediately! I was just appalled and, and hurt!" Dr. Oz wore a fat suit prosthesis which made him appear to weigh 400 pounds. This was his report. "Even though in my head I know I'm wearing a fat suit and I'm not really 400 pounds, my heart is saying, 'You're not worthy.'" He also reported feeling invisible when he wore the suit.

These celebrities are accustomed to eye contact and attention. What about the average Joe? Will wearing a fat suit prosthesis have the same effect? Researchers asked UCLA students with normal BMIs to wear fat suits as they moved around the campus (Incollingo Rodriguez et al., 2016). Other students were asked to wear the same clothing but without the fat suit as they walked around the campus. Then the students were asked to report their feelings. Did they feel angry, anxious, sad, hurt, or rejected while wearing the fat suit? The students reported more personal discomfort and negative feelings when wearing the suit. Later, the researchers asked the participants to select food and beverage rewards from an array. The students who had worn the fat suit selected and ate more unhealthy foods, and they consumed more calories.

Oldham et al. replicated these findings. They asked 120 people to wear a fat suit or control clothing in both public and private settings before offering them snack foods. Those wearing the body suits ate more snack foods. Women were more affected by the setting. They ate more snack foods if they had worn the fat suit in public (Oldham, Tomiyama, & Robinson, 2018).

These studies make four important points. Being judged by others as overweight is emotionally distressing and shaming. Second, being judged by others when you are overweight makes you eat more. Third, being judged as overweight makes you crave junk food. Finally, women are more vulnerable to the effects of being seen in public as overweight. Maybe that's why so many of us withdraw from social groups and stay at home with a tub of ice cream. Ice cream doesn't bite. People do.

Are you playing the shame game with your weight? There's a host of information on the Internet including worksheets and workbooks.

Shame, Cortisol, and the Brain

The negative effects of shame and stress on our weight is due to increased levels of cortisol. Cortisol is a glucocorticoid or steroid hormone produced by the adrenal gland. The importance of cortisol in the accumulation of body fat, particularly around the waist, was recognized when Cushing's Syndrome was identified. In Cushing's Syndrome, the adrenal gland produces too much cortisol, and the patient accumulates fat. The hypothalamic–pituitary–adrenocortical axis (HPA) responsible for controlling cortisol levels is illustrated in the figure. The brain structures involved are the hypothalamus and the anterior pituitary. Stress acts on the hypothalamus which produces the corticotropic releasing hormone (CRH). This hormone, in turn, stimulates the anterior pituitary. The anterior pituitary releases adrenocorticotropic hormone (ACTH) which stimulates the adrenal gland. The adrenal gland releases cortisol into the blood stream. When cortisol reaches the necessary level, the hypothalamus and anterior pituitary stop producing CRH and ACTH.

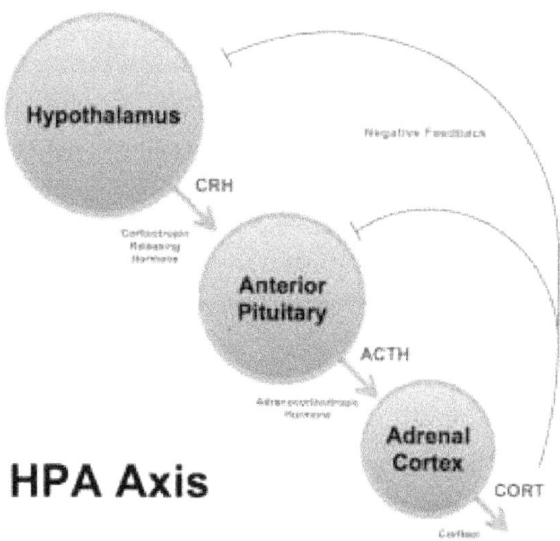

By BrianMSweis - Own work, CC BY-SA 3.0, https://commons.wikimedia.org/w/index.php?curid=23363130

Cortisol has many necessary and healthy functions, and the cortisol increases associated with normal life stresses are not harmful. However, prolonged high levels of cortisol are harmful. Dickerson et al. (2004) argue that of all the stressors you meet in your daily life, social situations which have the potential for negative judgment by others are "the most likely to engage the stress-responsive hypothalamic-pituitary-adrenocortical axis." The harm of sustained high cortisol levels is surprisingly far reaching. The harms include suppression of your immune system, high blood pressure, high blood sugar, insulin resistance, depression, poor planning and decision making, metabolic syndrome, Type II Diabetes, fat deposits on face, neck, and belly, reduced sex drive, bone loss, and carbohydrate cravings.

Now you can see why we wanted to talk about cortisol. Imagine this situation. An overweight man decides to lose weight, and he enrolls in a low-carbohydrate diet program. His marriage is failing, and his homelife is a misery. His job is high pressure, and his son was just arrested for dealing drugs. Will he lose weight? Probably not. His cortisol levels will pile the weight on even while he cuts down on carbs. He may then erroneously conclude that the diet program didn't work. Wrong. His life didn't work.

What does this suggest? Trying to lose weight when stress levels are out of control is damaging. Trying to lose weight under high stress conditions simply adds more pounds and makes us feel even more helpless.

How Does Cortisol Make Us Fat?

Janet Tomiyama and colleagues have developed a simple and useful model to answer this question (Tomiyama, 2014). The model involves four steps. When you become overweight, you experience social stigmatization and a variety of stresses associated with your weight. This stress acts on the HPA axis, and cortisol is released into the blood stream. The increased cortisol in your body stores more fat. The new pounds increase the stress level, and the cycle goes around, and around, and around.

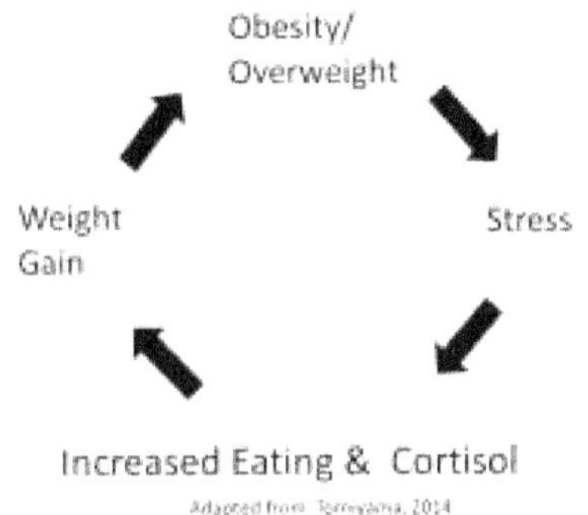

Let's look at the stress component of this model. Does stress increase eating? If so, how? There's a lot of information on this part of the model. This is really evidence for what we lay folks already know. We call it comfort eating. We've all done it. I can't count the number of times I've sent my husband to the store to buy ice cream or chocolate when I've felt down. Since I've given up most carbohydrates, particularly sugar, there have been no late night, "Honey would you get me some ice cream" requests.

The classic image of a comfort eater is the performance of the actress Goldie Hawn in *Death Becomes Her*. After a so-called friend steals her boyfriend, the main character (Hawn) locks herself in her apartment and stuffs herself with sweets and carbs until she is hugely overweight and forced into a hospital. Like the character in the movie, we overeat when we are depressed and anxious.

These moods are stressful, and they increase cortisol in our blood streams (Adam & Epel, 2017; Greeno & Wing, 1994). Stress makes us switch our food preferences from a normal diet to a diet filled with high fat and high sugar comfort foods (Epel, Lapidus, McEwen, & Brownell, 2001; Epel & Tomiyama, 2012; Pecoraro, Reyes, Gomez, Bhargava, & Dallman, 2004)

There are several studies showing that weight stigmatization makes us fat (Major, Eliezer, & Rieck, 2012; Schvey, Puhl, & Brownell, 2014; Tomiyama & Mann, 2013). Major et al. asked women to read an article about overweight individuals being stigmatized on the job because of their weight or a neutral article. Women who viewed themselves as overweight (even if they were lean) ate more calories after reading the article about weight discrimination in employment. Their blood pressures also rose. Schvey et al. (2014) asked overweight women to watch a weight stigmatizing video. They ate more calories after viewing the film than those women who'd just seen a neutral video.

Stress associated with being overweight and stigmatized not only makes us eat, but it changes the cortisol levels in our blood stream. Researchers looked at the changes in cortisol levels in the saliva of women who had viewed a ten-minute weight-stigmatizing video versus a neutral video (Schvey et al., 2014). The weight stigmatizing video was made up of clips which presented overweight women in pejorative ways such as overeating, wearing ill-fitting clothing, dancing in a comical manner, or trying to exercise. One representative clip showed an actress in a fat suit dancing in front of a group of male construction workers. The construction workers appear to be repulsed. Another clip shows a heavy woman trying on many pairs of trousers without success. The neutral clips were television commercials, bits from documentaries, etc. As the researchers expected, watching the weight-stigmatizing video clips increased cortisol in the saliva.

Watching videos making fun of overweight women was upsetting to all women, both overweight and lean. Take heed! Don't watch videos of fat people who are being used as comedic tools. It's bad for you, and it interferes with your ability to lose weight.

You might think we're going a bit overboard. The increases in cortisol won't last very long. You're wrong. These changes in cortisol levels have long-lasting effects. High cortisol levels make us hungry, and we eat. Cortisol also desensitizes the food reward system in the same way as sugar does (Adam & Epel, 2017; Rudenga & Small, 2012). That is, cortisol makes us hungry now and primes us to be hungry later. Research shows that people given a dose of glucocorticoid not only eat more immediately after exposure to cortisol, but they eat more later (Adam et al., 2010).

Shame and Weight Loss

What happens when you diet but don't lose weight? You feel shame. As you just learned, being ashamed triggers cortisol release. Shame also plays another nasty trick. It makes you more self-conscious about your weight and more vulnerable to stigmatization. You begin to actively search for shaming events, threats, and ridicule (Kaiser, Vick, & Major, 2006).

Two recent papers show how experiencing stigmatization about your weight increases your risk of remaining overweight or even gaining pounds in the long run. In a national sample of over 6,000 people, Sutin and Terracciano found that lean participants who'd experienced weight discrimination were 2.5 times more likely to be obese at a four-year follow-up than those not experiencing discrimination (Sutin & Terracciano, 2013). The effect was larger when the individual was already struggling with weight stigmatization. In an adolescent sample of over 2,000 girls, investigators found that girls who were labeled as "too fat" by age 10 were 1.7 times more likely to be obese at 19 compared to those who were not labeled as too fat (Hunger & Tomiyama, 2014).

Please, don't tell anyone they're fat, particularly a child. Ban fat jokes. Don't let anyone else make jokes or tell a child they're fat either!

What to Do?

Evaluate your sense of comradery with other people struggling with their weights. Most groups band together when they face discrimination. They find people in their group to admire and emulate. Overweight people, on the other hand, tend to withdraw into their shells. They find few role models to look up to. You might want to look at the fat acceptance movement. See the book by Linda Bacon, Ph.D., *Health at Every Size: The Surprising Truth About Your Weight* (Bacon, 2008). This book may help you set realistic goals for your health and secondarily for your weight. Follow the blogs of positive role models such as Your Fat Friend. https://medium.com/@thefatshadow

Get wild. Start a blog of your own.

Evaluate the impact that your friends and family have on your emotions. We hate to say this, but the greatest stigmatizers and barriers to our success are most often the people who say they love us unconditionally—our families and our friends (Puhl, Himmelstein, & Quinn, 2018).

we're reminded of a lovely woman we once knew. She had gained weight after the births of her four children, and her husband started nagging her about her weight. She decided to lose weight, and she did. As the pounds dropped off, her husband became increasingly jealous. He believed that she was losing weight so that she could have an affair and leave him. As you might guess, their marriage was doomed. Losing weight made her realize that her husband was not on her team. Rather, he was a stressor, a source of unhappiness. Another friend had a very bad eating day after a mutual friend said with a sigh while looking at her belly, "You have such a pretty face." The implication was the rest of her wasn't pretty at all.

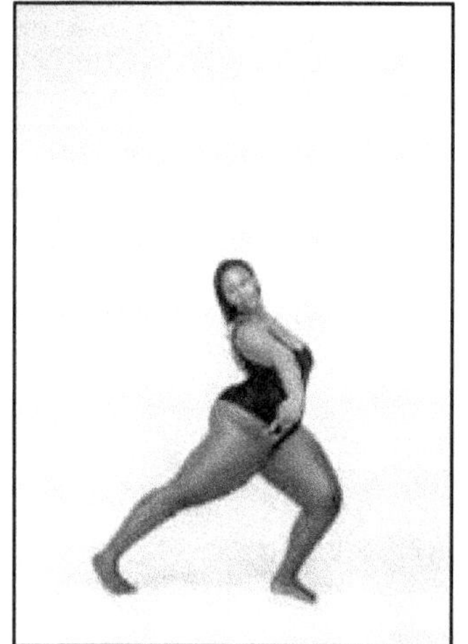

Take a long hard look at the stress inducing and stigmatizing people in your life. Get rid of them. Don't declutter your house, declutter your life.

Find your anger. We're going to keep hammering on this until you get it. We like the words of an in-your-face mama, Laura Beck. This is what she wrote about celebrities wearing fat suits. "My body is not a joke, and when you act like it is, you are a terrible, shitty garbage person who is actively participating in the objectification of women." She describes herself as a "Real Life Fat Woman" or RLFW. She encourages you to get going and to make use of the anger we know, and she knows, you've locked somewhere deep in your soul.

Self-acceptance can reduce stress and help us lose weight. This woman is proud of her body and her size. Photo by Jennifer Enujiugha from Pexels. Take a look at the Health-At-Every Size (HAES) movement and their approach to weight management (Bacon et al., 2002; Provencher et al., 2009).

The HAES tenants are the following:

- Accept your size.
- Trust yourself.
- Adopt healthy lifestyle habits by finding the joy in your life, eat when you're hungry, and tailor your tastes to enjoy nutritious foods.
- Embrace size diversity.

Don't try losing weight alone. Find someone to share the highs and lows of the journey. I benefited from the suggestions of my weight loss counselor, Barb. She's a special person who lost 95 pounds. She is knowledgeable and caring. Make sure you have a competent advisor. Sadly, the people you trust to guide your health decisions (doctors, therapists, etc.) sometimes look down on you because you're overweight. There is a shocking bias among healthcare workers against overweight and obese patients (Wimalawansa, 2014). Healthcare providers sometimes see their overweight patients as unattractive and having poor self-esteem. Nurses and therapists also have negative biases toward overweight patients, stereotyping them as lazy, lacking in self-control, and noncompliant.

Frankly, many medical practitioners don't know what to do with you. That's because medical training doesn't emphasize nutrition. See discussion by Debra Minger in her book, *Death by Food Pyramid* (Minger, 2007).

There are lots of good competent people who will be glad to help you, and there's no reason to be stuck with a snake oil salesman.

Exercises

1. How much self-blaming do you do? When you have negative thoughts, tell them, "Stop." The negative thoughts will return, but they're weaker each time.
2. Build a support team that knows what they're talking about.
3. Make a list of your critical, unsympathetic family members and friends. Make a pledge. Don't listen to them. Remember, their negativity goes straight to your brain and grows roots there.

CHAPTER 16

I like rice. Rice is great if you're hungry and want to eat a thousand of something. — Mitch Hedberg

Ready, Set, Go

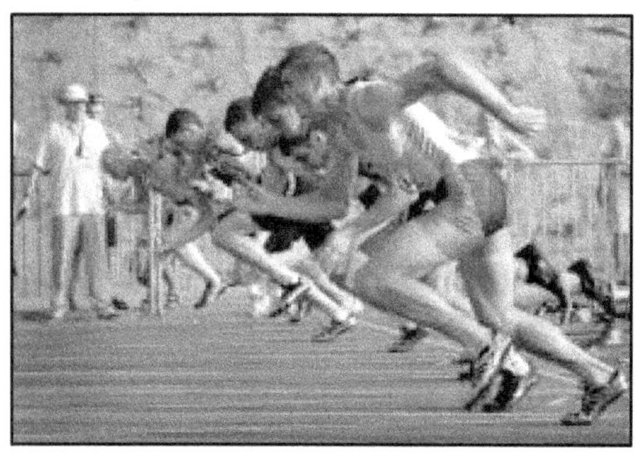

Do you make New Year's Resolutions? How many of these resolutions involved eating a healthier diet and exercising more? Marketing experts know we make these silly resolutions year after year. Throughout the month of January, advertisers bombard us with special dietary products, vitamins, food plans, and exercise machines. They tell us to act now and save money. Photo /www.pexels.com/photo/athletes-running-on-track-and-field-oval-in-grayscale-photography-34514/

You won't lose weight because you have an exercise machine stored under your bed or in the den. The ignored supplement bottles on your shelf won't make you lose weight. You'll lose weight because you follow up your decision to lose weight with a plan—not a purchase, but a plan. The planning stage is critical to successful weight loss. Good planning is the watershed of any weight loss program.

* * * *

My weight loss journey started in January in a typical way. I said to my belly, "Whew, the holidays are over, and now I can get those pounds off." I literally wandered into the Metabolic Research Center™ feeling totally lost and without direction. Fortunately, the MRC program gave me the direction I needed.

Early in the book, I declared that I am a carbohydrate addict. I did this for a purpose. You have a disease. I have a disease. Our illness is chronic. It won't go away. If you cling to the hope that you can go back to your old familiar way of eating when the initial weight loss phase ends, you're wrong. You may think that this phase is behind you, but it isn't. Eating to excess is like any other chronic illness. We must manage it in the same way. If you have a low thyroid level, you don't stop taking your thyroid replacement medication simply because some lab results came back normal. We want you to be successful, but we want you to appreciate the nature of your adversary as we contemplate a weight loss plan.

History Is Everything

Your weight history will tell you what your weight loss time frame will be. Will it take you six months of active weight loss strategies combined with one year follow up to maintain your gains? Will you require a longer time frame? Will you need to divide your weight loss plan into segments with a maintenance phase in between?

For many of us, our belly fat has been keeping us company for a very long time. In general, the longer your belly fat has been with you, the more time it will take to lose weight and to reset your body's metabolism. Based on an average of three pounds of weight loss every two weeks, it could take a year to lose 66 pounds, two years to lose 132 pounds (Teixeira et al., 2002). That's the optimistic range for weight loss during a weight loss program. If your weight loss rate is less than one pound per week, it will take you twice as long to reach these numbers.

A high BMI in childhood leading to an overweight adult is much harder to reverse. This makes a kind of sense. If you believe the research, as we do, your brain and metabolism are set by age five (Hemmingsson, 2018). Retraining your habits and your metabolism will take longer for you than for someone who was once lean and became overweight as an adult.

Yo-Yo Weight Loss

Are you a cyclic or chronic dieter? Would you describe yourself as a Yo-Yo dieter? This term was coined by Kelly Brownell to describe cyclical weight gain, loss, and regain—akin to the up-and down-motion of a Yo-Yo (Rhee, 2017). Do you believe that you gain back more weight each time you diet? That is, your starting weight was 170 on cycle 1, you dropped back to 145, and regained the weight plus a few more pounds to 180. Do you believe that this weight cycling is bad for your health? Have you been advised that it's better to stay overweight than to risk the Yo-Yo?

You won't be alone if you said yes to these questions. The popular wisdom that weight cycling is bad for your health is unsupported by science. These beliefs about the effects of Yo-Yo dieting are so firmly entrenched that they've achieved the status of facts (Palm, Schram, Swarts, van Schothorst, & Keijer, 2017). Although many studies don't allow firm conclusions about the metabolic and health consequences of Yo-Yo dieting, the best of the best studies tell us that Yo-Yo dieting does not necessarily lead to increased weight gain, diabetes, serious illness, or death (El Ghoch, Calugi, & Dalle Grave, 2018; Mackie, Samocha-Bonet, & Tam, 2017; Palm et al., 2017). There's some early evidence that losing weight, even if we regain some or all of it, may improve our metabolic health (Palm et al., 2017).

There's one exception. If you have fragile health, all weight loss programs are stressful. There is evidence suggesting an increased risk of cardiovascular problems such as high blood pressure after Yo-Yo dieting (Rhee, 2017).

If you've experienced a weight regain after a weight loss attempt, there are two possible explanations. First, most dieters drastically change the macronutrient composition of their diets when trying to lose weight (Palm et al., 2017). If the foods on your diet are unhealthy and lack enough nutrients, the body may be set to rebuild itself with a vengeance. Second, the weight gain of a Yo-Yo is depressing. We regain weight, become depressed and discouraged. We eat fat and sugar laden foods to comfort ourselves (Madigan, Pavey, Daley, Jolly, & Brown, 2018).

Celebrate Failed Weight Loss Attempts

You may be asking yourself if we've gone off the deep end. We haven't. Unsuccessful attempts to lose weight are a cause for celebration. Let's find out why.

The three psychological dimensions of eating are restrained eating, emotional eating, and external eating (Elfhag & Morey, 2008). Emotional eating means you are inclined to eat in response to negative emotions such as depression, disappointment, or feelings of loneliness. That is, you feel sad, you eat pie. External eating means you eat in response to external food cues such as the sight, smell, and taste of food. You see a half-eaten bag of chocolate in your pantry, and you eat it. You weren't thinking about the chocolate until you saw it. Emotional and external eating are problematic eating behaviors.

Restrained eating, on the other hand, is a strength because it requires conscious determination and effort to restrict your food intake and calories. If you have dieted and lost weight, you have restrained eating skills. Individuals with a history of restrained eating are more likely to reach their weight loss goals (James et al., 2018). However, those of us with many failed weight loss attempts are more likely to drop out of a weight loss program (Horstmann et al., 2015; Hulbert-Williams et al., 2017; James et al., 2018; J. Teixeira et al., 2002; P. J. Teixeira, Palmeira, et al., 2004).

How do we reconcile these apparently contradictory findings? We think emotional variables explain the difference. If we have a long history of failed weight loss attempts, we are more likely to see any bump in the road as indicating the current weight loss effort is doomed. We forget to give ourselves credit for what we have accomplished and focus instead on what we didn't.

We must reframe Yo-Yo dieting from a negative to a positive. We suggest that it's better to have dieted and lost then to have never dieted at all. If we don't let ourselves become overwhelmed by failed weight loss attempts, we can learn from each diet experience. First, be proud of yourself. You chose to diet. You did diet. You lost weight. This means you have useful skills. You probably just ate the wrong combination and amounts of foods.

This was my experience. I set up a food program and followed it. I basically cut back on calories. I ate the same mix of foods, but I ate smaller amounts. I couldn't maintain the weight I lost. My first mistake was to blame myself. I had failed. Wrong. Evidence shows that our ability to be a restrained or controlled eater gets better with time and practice. When I identified my carbohydrate addiction and cut back on carbs, I was able to meet my weight loss goal. I had the skills. I had simply followed the wrong diet.

If you berate yourself as I did for failing, you've made a serious mistake. You only fail if you keep repeating the same mistake. "The definition of insanity is doing the same thing over and over but expecting different results."— A. Einstein

Practice Joy

Starting your diet with a grim sense of determination may help you get going, but this attitude won't help you deal with the ups and the downs of the diet process. Flexibility and joy are the keys. Look at your upcoming weight loss attempt with anticipation not dread. We promise you it will be a learning experience, and you will benefit from it no matter how many pounds you lose.

Most writers agree that close adherence to your diet during the early phases of weight loss is essential. If the plan says four ounces, get out your scale and measure your portion before you eat it. Seek consultation before you tinker with your plan. Don't change it on your own. That means for the first month or two you must stick to the diet. However, when you're losing weight each week, you can and should be more flexible.

Any weight loss program will require a drastic reduction in refined sugar and starch consumption. If you adopt a scorched earth policy—no sugar absolutely no sugar ever—you're more likely to collapse and start eating every sugar in sight. If you use flexible restraint and allow yourself to enjoy favorite treats, you're more likely to succeed in changing your food preference away from high glycemic index foods like sugar and toward foods with lower glycemic indices like fruit (James et al., 2018). It's okay, and even good, to break from your plan and include favorite foods. Plan your treat. For example, my favorite birthday cake is chocolate on chocolate. I bought two pieces of incredibly decadent chocolate cake, and I enjoyed every morsel. I didn't gain an ounce. I did, however, experience a resurgence of cravings. If your cravings are irresistible after a treat, you will have to stick closely to your plan for a bit longer before adding a treat.

Develop a Weight Loss Team

Nothing is more important than your weight loss team. That's right, team. Countless studies have demonstrated the necessity of social support for weight loss. Let's look at some of the research. First, many of us get discouraged during the early weeks of weight loss. The excitement of a new challenge fades.

Those who get social support during the early weeks are less likely to drop out (Polk et al., 2017). Second, education is essential. You may think you know all there is to know about weight loss, but you don't. I discovered that losing weight was a very intense and sometimes disturbing emotional experience. It was lifesaving to have a counselor to help, educate, and encourage.

Your first diet program may not work. It is here that a knowledgeable counselor is essential. Your program must be tweaked and adjusted on a weekly basis for the first two to three months. If you don't make the right adjustments, weight loss stalls, you get discouraged, and you quit. Without my counselor's input, I wouldn't have known how to adjust my diet. I particularly struggled with the increased fat and protein requirements of my diet plan.

The support (or at the very least cooperation) of the people around you can be helpful if it's the right kind of support (Karfopoulou, Anastasiou, Avgeraki, Kosmidis, & Yannakoulia, 2016). Encouragement and compliments are helpful. Instruction is not helpful. If those supporting you want to take over a therapeutic role, explain that what you need is a cheerleader not another weight loss counselor. Research shows that a couple who diets together, loses weight together. Encourage, but don't browbeat, those in your household to join you if they are also struggling with weight issues.

Before you start dieting, send up some test balloons. Describe what you're planning to friends and family. Get their reactions. Recognize when you are becoming an outlier in their eyes and when your diet process will challenge what those around you see as normal.

Set Weight Loss Goals with Care

This is another important aspect of developing a successful weight loss plan. After I'd enrolled in the weight loss program, Barb asked me to set a target weight. I wasn't sure what to select because my weight had ranged more than 50 pounds over the years. I decided on the middle ground. To my surprise, I lost more weight than I'd expected. In fact, by following the diet, I dropped to a weight I hadn't remotely considered. The weight my body selected came as a complete surprise to the conscious me.

Your body has a weight goal of its own. You can't let your idea of the right weight set you up to fight your body. If you set your weight goal too low, your weight loss will stall above your desired weight. This will make you unhappy. Then, of course, the old failure monster rears its ugly head. Try this first. Set an initial weight which would make you happy. This should be a modest goal.

Second, decide on your ideal weight. Third, calculate how long it will take to reach each goal (use a metric of 1 to 1.5 pounds per week). Finally, give your body permission to decide on your final weight. If you go too low, you risk a rapid weight regain. If you can't accept giving control to your body, you may have an eating disorder. You will need the support of a counselor to overcome this.

Know Where the Tiger Has Its Lair

The tiger is giving up on your weight loss plan. Giving up is more likely to occur in the first three months of a diet (Sawamoto, 2015). At least 30% of weight loss clients drop out during these months.

Don't set yourself up to fail by starting a diet in November. Do you really think you can make it through the November and December socially mandated food orgies without giving in? Don't start a weight loss plan before a very stressful event or important family holiday. Pick the best starting time you can.

People who can't keep up with the schedule of meetings and appointments are more likely to drop out of weight loss programs (Teixeira et al., 2002). People don't stop coming to sessions because they no longer wish to lose weight. They stop attending because something in their lives got in the way and took precedence. Regular meetings and weigh-ins are essential to long-term success.

We were saddened by a recent Nutrisystem commercial. Lovely Marie Osmond says, "Count, measure, meetings? Not with Nutrisystem." Marie is telling us that we don't need any of that awful stuff like weigh-ins or visits to the weight loss center. All you need is Nutrisystem products. Somehow, apparently by osmosis, you'll learn how to prepare and eat the correct amounts of foods. You're being advised to abandon the very things which will make you succeed in long-term weight loss.

Are You Ready?

How ready are you to begin a successful weight loss program? The first issue is choosing your weight loss program. There are lots of choices out there. If you're a carbohydrate addict and you've gotten this far in the book, we hope you've accepted the necessity for starting a low-carb diet. We'll go into the specifics of the diet in detail in the next chapter.

To help you assess your readiness to make a behavioral change, the readiness to change stages are presented in a chart (Zimmerman, Olsen, & Bosworth, 2000).

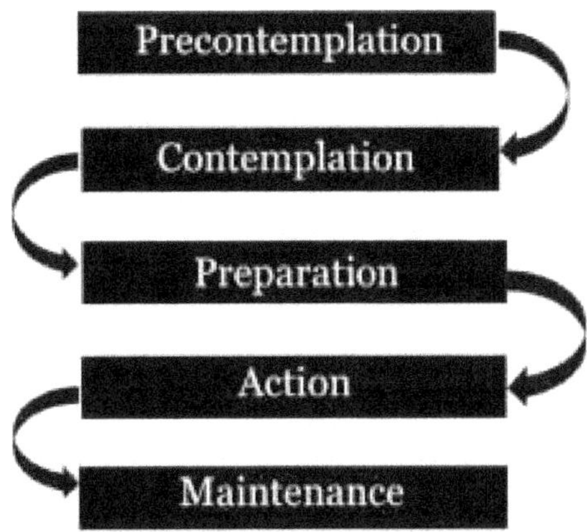

Adapted from Zimmerman et al., 2000

If you are in the precontemplation stage, you have no intention of embarking on a weight loss program within the near future. If you are reading this book, you've probably already completed this stage and are aware of your need to change your eating behavior.

If you are in the contemplation stage, you know that you have a weight problem and you're seriously thinking about overcoming it. However, you have not committed to any specific actions.

If you are in the preparation stage, you plan to act in the next month and you may have already made some small changes. Your actions have not, thus far, led to any significant weight loss.

If you're in the action stage, you are modifying your behavior and environment to overcome your weight problem. These actions require a considerable commitment of time and energy. If you have successfully altered your dysfunctional eating pattern for a period of one day to six months, you are in this stage.

If you're in the maintenance stage, you are working to prevent relapse and to consolidate the gains you've made. The maintenance stage lasts from six months to an indeterminate period past the initial action. Maintaining weight loss is the most challenging stage. I'm still trying to figure it out.

The stages must be viewed as a process. We don't necessarily go through the stages in the same order or at the same rates. You must expect that you could fall back on old eating patterns and have to repeat some of the stages. Some experts say that the stages shouldn't be viewed as linear, but rather, as a spiral. Returning to a previous stage is normal and not a defeat. Let's say, you take action and begin a weight loss program, but you don't lose weight. When you examine your reasons for ending your plan, you'll probably discover that you weren't adequately prepared. You shouldn't give up, but you should go back to the preparation stage, rethink your plan, and begin again.

We won't go into detail about the preparation needed before you start your weight loss program because other authors have provided good suggestions. Dr. Ludwig suggests a 7-day countdown for the week prior to beginning your diet. See Dr. Ludwig's book, *Always Hungry* for more information (Ludwig, 2016). See our modification of Dr. Ludwig's countdown.

Day 1. Familiarize yourself with the nutritional goals of your weight loss program.

Day 2. Take a health snapshot and start tracking. Collect your baseline weight data and start paying attention to what you eat. Don't change anything, just observe. Your weight loss counselor will help you with this.

Day 3. Look at your sleep, activity and stress relief strategies. Do you have any issues with these? Do you have any solutions? Make a note if you don't have a solution and be prepared to talk to your counselor.

Day 4. Decide on your weight loss goals. Choose a happy weight and an ideal weight. How will you deal with relapses or deviations from your diet plan? How will you get back on track?

Day 5. Prepare your home and kitchen for a new way of eating. For example, do you need to get an air fryer to cook fried foods? Do you need insulated bags to carry foods to work for lunch? Dispose of foods in cupboards and refrigerator which don't fit with your diet plan. This was hard for me. I hate to throw anything away, but I also know that I'm very cue dominated. I can't have chocolate, candy, or doughnuts in the house. I will eat them. All of them!

Day 6. Go shopping. Restock your refrigerator and cupboards with foods required for the low-carb diet.

Day 7. Make a menu plan for the first week. If possible, make a dish that will last all or most of the week. Soups, roasts, etc. are good evening meal choices. That gives you fewer choices to face each day. We make approximately 200 food choices each day. We find this number incredible, but experts say it's true.

Exercises

1.   Think of how good it will feel to succeed.
2.   Watch a funny movie or do something that makes you laugh.

CHAPTER 17

He who does not mind his belly, will hardly mind anything else.
— Samuel Johnson

Get Rid of Caroline or Bust!

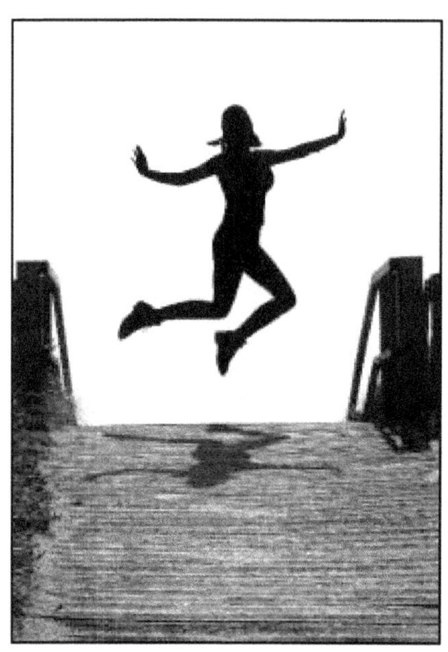

There's nothing harder than changing the way you live. We develop very deep affections for our way of doing things. Even though we sometimes desire change, we want to order those changes just like we order takeout meals. I was nervous, very nervous, when I started my diet. I wondered the night before I started, the day I went to the weight loss clinic, and many times during the first week of my diet. Had I made a mistake?

Image by <a ref="https://pixabay.com/users/Anemone123-2637160/

*** * * ***

On our initial weigh-in, my weight loss counselor asked a critical question, one which I found surprisingly difficult to answer: "What is your problem food?" I thought for a moment before answering, "chocolate". As you will see, chocolate is not my problem food. By problem food, I mean the food which supports or fuels your carbohydrate addiction. I didn't know what my problem food was. You might not know what your problem food is either. Then, we set my weight loss goal. I had a modest goal. I'd always been comfortable when I weighed about 142 pounds. I selected this as my goal.

Next, she took body measurements, every part of me. To make matters worse, she added up the numbers. I added up to 338.75 inches. Next, she weighed me on a scale which calculated body fat. I didn't want to face my enemy. I'd avoided scales and mirrors. I wasn't happy with the weight she recorded. I liked my body fat numbers even less. My body was made up of 42.4% fat! After the measurements, she gave me a meal handout, a chart to write down the foods I'd eaten, and a bag of supplements. I tried to absorb the bad news. I had to weigh my food, and I couldn't eat carbohydrates for two weeks. After the two weeks, I could have one carbohydrate per day (equivalent to one slice of bread). My counselor explained that I'd committed to a lifestyle change. This wasn't a short-term program to follow until I got the pounds off. This was for always. I'd made a commitment to my health. I pushed my fears and doubts aside. I was going to play this one by the rules.

I didn't own a food scale, so I bought one on the way home. I stopped at the grocery and stocked up on produce. I passed up the fruit, bakery, and chip sections with a real sense of loss. I would be able to eat small amounts of fruits, but I had to view chips and bakery products as toxic.

I had carbohydrates galore at home. There was no way I would stick to the no carbohydrate rule with them still in the house singing to me like the sirens sang to Ulysses. Thus began the great purge. I was relentless. I pulled boxes and jars from every nook and cranny in the house. I said a lingering goodbye to my last six pack of Coca Cola. I'd learned to love this stuff in my teens. One by one I looked at the labels of foods in my pantry. I was shocked. The jar of spaghetti sauce contained many carbohydrates. Ketchup also has sugar. There were carbohydrates in my bottled salad dressings. These dressings had to go. I read the label on my breakfast cereal—loaded with carbohydrates. Out it went. In fact, I was finding little on my shelves that didn't include sugar. I realized that I had to toss all boxes except for a few basics (I did keep the ketchup).

I had to deal with my baking and cooking supplies. I had stashes of flour, white sugar, corn syrup, molasses, beans, every pasta ever invented, honey, etc. It took extra control to toss jars of apple sauce, jam, and maple syrup. It's funny how deep certain foods go to the roots of our psyches. Tossing out the jar of maple syrup was agony because this act meant that I'd eaten my last pancake or piece of French toast. I love pasta. Now, it is on the forbidden list. When I'd finished, my pantry was bare. Then I looked in the refrigerator. I read the labels of the bottles and containers. The frozen orange juice had to go. No more processed fruit drinks. Too much sugar. I pulled the low-fat milk from the shelf and read the label. My low-fat milk had no fat, but it had many carbohydrates. I later learned that the milk processors had pulled every bit of fat out of milk and left the carbohydrates. They then added some vitamins and nutrients back in. The milk went down the drain. Back to the store to buy whole milk. I felt almost indecent carrying a carton of fat laced whole milk when we checked out.

With my pantry and refrigerator cleared of temptations, I read through the diet sheet. It was overwhelming, and I felt slightly depressed. The program was telling me to eat a fat at each meal. After watching endless commercials on the dangers of high cholesterol, I'd spent countless hours trying to learn to cook without butter. I had learned to live without eggs. I had gotten used to skim milk and processed low fat spread with some considerable effort. Now, I was supposed to use real butter and whole milk. I was encouraged to eat eggs as a source of protein. I was getting a mild headache, and I felt a growing sense of irritation. Is our world crazy? I wished for something to believe in, to trust. Could I trust the low carbohydrate diet or was it another fad unsupported by science? I pushed these thoughts aside. Best get on to the task at hand. Study the diet. The program looked something like this:

- Eat three meals per day. Don't skip meals.
- Drink copious amounts of water to help move fat from storage (80 ounces or 10 glasses).
- Eat the following at each meal: A 4-ounce serving of healthy protein (lean meat or fish, cottage cheese, any variety of cheese, and up to three eggs); 4 ounces of cooked or 8 ounces of raw vegetables; and a fat (2 ounces of avocado, 1 tablespoon butter, ¼ cup olives, or 1 ounce of nuts, etc.)
- Weigh your foods.
- Take two proprietary supplements before each meal (combination of herbs to help with weight redistribution and curb appetite). Another supplement with each meal.
- Drink four clear protein drinks each day.

- Drink a supplement between meals to promote development of ketosis.
- No carbohydrates (bread, breakfast cereal, crackers, potatoes, and all baked goods). I love chocolate doughnuts. I said goodbye to them.
- No drinks containing carbohydrates. Another favorite taken away. I had congratulated myself on my nobility when I'd ordered a low-fat latte. Wrong again!

I found the diet more than a little overwhelming, and my brain couldn't contain all the information. I don't know if this was my resistance to change. I had to make a chart to keep track of all the supplements and drinks. I don't like lists and charts. This was becoming way too hard. There was a mounting sense of dread. Dieting always makes me feel awful. It takes a few days of reduced calories, but I always end up with a growling stomach, cravings, and nagging headaches. I have all this new diet stuff to deal with and pain to look forward to. It's too much. I decided to put off starting my diet until the following day. I pulled a bag of crackers from the trash and munched a few.

Day 1

I'll never forget my first low carb meal. It's etched on my memory in indelible ink. First, I had my supplements. I had to take these to curb my appetite. Then, I had three scrambled eggs, a slice of avocado, and a large salad. I hadn't eaten three eggs at one sitting in years. Once after a doctor-induced cholesterol panic, I didn't eat an egg for an entire year. The salad was huge, and it was disturbingly unnatural to eat salad for breakfast. Don't get me wrong, I like salads. Eggs are supposed to be accompanied by a piece of toast, not a salad. I then drank a glass of protein drink (clear and no carbohydrates). I was stuffed. I couldn't eat another morsel. According to my schedule, I was to have a mid-morning drink. I was in no mood for more intake, but I was determined to follow the rules.

I knew one thing for sure—I needed help. I needed to accept the wisdom of others. This was hard for me as I tend to think of myself as a critical thinker—a nice way of saying I go against authority. I plunged onward. Lunch was low-fat cottage cheese and another gigantic salad. Of course, there were supplements, water, and protein drinks. My mid-afternoon keto-stimulating drink was followed by a small steak and more salad. Boy did I miss the baked potato. More supplements.

Day 1 of my diet program provided my first lesson, one which I suspect many of you will share. I discovered the strength of my cultural food conditioning. "Salads are not breakfast foods," the old me said. The new me is starting to enjoy salad for breakfast. When you think about it, there's no reason why we can't eat a salad or any other food for breakfast or any other meal, but that's not how it feels. We're overweight because we follow our cultural conditioning. Channel the rebel in your psyche and resist because much of our conditioning is unhealthy.

First Weigh-In

By the end of the first week, I'd memorized the diet plan, and I'd accepted the necessity of measuring my food portions. I learned during the first week that I couldn't estimate food quantities accurately. I realized that this probably contributed to my weight problem. I wasn't realistic about how much I was eating. I felt a mild sense of pride. I had stuck to the program as written. I had learned one cause of my weight problem—my food quantities were too large. I put my dinner plate away and now eat from a salad plate.

I was afraid to weigh myself, so I went to my weigh-in with a sense of anxiety. I didn't expect much. I'd been putting stuff in my mouth at a high rate for a week. What happened? I'd lost 2.6 pounds! I'd lost weight, and I hadn't felt hungry. No headaches. No growling stomach. I'd felt full. I did notice a little nausea. I learned that this reaction was common. To the lay public, it's called the keto flu. Not everyone gets keto flu, but I learned these mild symptoms were temporary. They had something to do with the body switching over from a glucose–based metabolism to ketosis.

I left the weight loss center wanting to giggle and sing. How was it possible to eat fat, feel full, and lose weight? Certainly, something was wrong here. My dark side argued, "probably too good to last."

Second Weigh-In

The second session also stands out. I'd lost another 2.4 pounds. I'd never lost this much weight in two weeks. I discussed how comfortable this diet was with Barb. I didn't experience pain other than a very mild case of keto flu. I asked why? Barb explained that fat and protein make you feel full, but carbs make you feel hungry and induce cravings. Often, we follow a calorie counting approach when we try to lose weight. In this model, we cut back fats, proteins, and carbohydrates. When we keep carbohydrates in our diets, we don't have enough fat and protein to counterbalance their effect on hunger. Thus, we feel pain. When we eat enough proteins and fats but no carbohydrates, we don't experience as much hunger.

On day 10, I had the vivid cake dream I described earlier. I was also having waking cravings. I walked past the cookie section of the market. The cookies were talking to me. I could smell them through their packages. I managed to get by the temptations, but I decided that I had to stay out of those aisles. I had nearly yielded to a craving. These experiences made me consider the possibility that I had a carbohydrate addiction. I discussed the idea of carb addiction with Barb. She described her lengthy struggle with weight. She had become a diet expert. She had tried literally everything. It was only when she stopped eating carbs that she lost weight and maintained her weight loss. She suggested that I wasn't addicted to food or eating, but I was addicted to carbs.

This was a big week for me. I got to eat a small amount of carbohydrates each day. Wow! I added an apple to my menu.

Third Weigh In

The mild stomach distress and flu-like symptoms of week 1 and 2 decreased. My first real health payoff came during the third week. My symptoms of gastric reflux disease (GERD) were reduced. I had taken medication for GERD for more years than I liked to think about. I'd tried several dietary approaches with no success. When I removed sugar from my diet, my reflux symptoms were reduced. I stopped taking medication.

I'd learned a very important truth. Sugar in the stomach makes acid, acid makes pain and reflux. When I looked back, I remembered that I always had terrible reflux symptoms when I went out to dinner. At these meals, I always drank wine and maybe a mixed drink, and I always had dessert. I blamed the fat, but I never considered the carbohydrates I'd consumed.

Sadly, the health benefits I was experiencing on the diet were counterbalanced by the 1.8 pounds I'd gained. I'd stayed true to the diet with no lapses. Why had I gained weight? After reviewing my meals, Barb suggested that the added apple with its carbohydrates was the culprit. In her experience, some clients are more vulnerable to carbohydrates than others. These individuals (count me in) gain weight if you wave a chocolate muffin in their general direction. Others can eat a few carbohydrates and stay in control of their weight. The other possibility was the amount of protein I was consuming. I decided to cut back protein intake by 1/3, and I decided to stay off carbohydrates indefinitely. No more apples!

I'd learned two more truths. First, I am vulnerable to carbohydrate consumption. My body latches onto carbohydrates and turns them into fat with ridiculous efficiency.

Second, successful weight loss requires ongoing adjustments. I was learning that you must tinker with your diet repeatedly to continue losing weight. This is hard to do without a competent counselor to suggest reasons why your weight loss rate has changed.

Fourth Weigh-In

Dropping the daily carbohydrate and decreasing the amount of protein by 1/3 worked. My weight loss was back on track. I hadn't experienced the increased energy that some dieters report, but I was happy with the all-important lower readings on the scale. I felt confident. I understood the diet, and the diet was working better. I had lost three more pounds. I'd lost weight faster and easier than any previous diet attempt.

Another health benefit emerged at the end of the first month. I had constipation issues for many years. This annoying problem was gone, gone, gone! Barb explained that your gastrointestinal health is improved on the ketogenic diet (something to do with bacteria in the gut).

I was also experiencing strange surges of emotion. I was near euphoria on some days, but I felt low and sluggish on other days. Some days I felt very, very angry. These strong emotions were not the result of keto flu. My body had adjusted to a ketogenic diet. Why these emotions? Other diets made me depressed, but I had never been emotionally volatile. I looked to the Internet to explain my reactions. I could find no information, nothing. All I could find on the Internet were personal stories about how terrific people felt on the diet or stories about the diet not working or being dangerous. I did a deeper search to find books related to the psychology of eating. I found four books that were vaguely related to my experiences.

When I read about other addictions (e.g., drugs and gaming), there were discussions about the emotional aspects which cause the addictive disorders as well as considerations of the emotional problems which occur during withdrawal from the substance or activity. Why was there no mention of the emotions linked to carbohydrate addiction? I don't know why we don't talk about the emotional aspects of carbohydrate addiction, but we simply don't.

From the other addictions, we know that treating these emotional reactions and their underpinnings is essential to treatment success. I decided to search the professional literature to find studies related to emotion and overeating and to try and synthesize them in a way which might be helpful to my sister and brother carbohydrate addicts.

Incidentally, Robert and I eat our meals together, so my diet became his diet. He started to lose weight as well.

Fifth to Tenth Weigh-Ins

I lost another 1.2 pounds before the fifth weigh-in. By the sixth weigh-in, I'd lost another 3.4 pounds. Barb pointed out that Caroline (my belly fat) was smaller. I ventured a peek into a mirror. She was right. Caroline was still there, but she was decidedly smaller.

During the next few weeks, I stuck to the diet, and I continued to lose weight in the following sequence: Week 7 = 3.0 pounds; week 8 = 1.2 pounds; week 9 = 5 pounds; week 10 = .6 pounds.

Time for a shopping trip. My first shopping trip since I'd started the ketogenic diet was a delight. I had lost one size. I bought a new pair of trousers to celebrate. I could have danced out of the department store.

My first big relapse. I was feeling pretty smug by this time. I'd reached my target weight, and I'd been a very good girl. I had stuck to my diet with no lapses. I felt strong and invulnerable. After my weigh-in, I decided to celebrate with a little of my favorite addictive substance, chocolate. I headed to an upscale market which carries quality foods. No food chain major brand candy bars for me. I wanted something exotic, something worthy of a celebration. My first mistake was wandering into the bakery. They had free samples of cookies and cake. I thought, "No problem having a few samples." I pulled myself away from the bakery and walked the aisles searching for a "healthy chocolate." I chose a bag of chocolate covered mangoes. I planned to eat four or five pieces each day. Was I ever living in a delusion! I took my prize to my car and opened it. I ate the candy pieces as I drove home. By the time I reached home, I'd eaten half the bag. Getting home brought me out of my sugar daze, and I tucked the package into the pantry. I thought I was done, but I wasn't. I couldn't put the chocolate out of my mind. I submitted. I caved. I ate the rest of the bag.

I was getting tired of learning lessons by this time, but this lesson couldn't be avoided. I wasn't strong when it came to chocolate. My diet hadn't cured my addiction. I am extremely susceptible to eating even one sugary carbohydrate. Eating one leads to eating another, and so on. I cannot keep contracts I make with myself when it comes to carbohydrates. For me, abstinence and avoidance of exposure to carbohydrates are essential if I am to maintain my weight loss. When it comes to carbohydrates, I am like the fire horse of yore. One ring of the bell, and I'm off.

Sessions 11 to 24

To my delight, I stuck with my diet, and I continued to lose weight. The number of pounds lost varied from .6 to 3.2 pounds per week. I was shocked when I reached my college weight. I was now two sizes smaller than when I started. Few of my clothes fit any more including bathing suits and underwear. I was a little nervous. Would I continue to lose and lose weight until I disappeared like the Cheshire cat, leaving only my smile behind? The answer to my worry was "no".

At the 21st weigh-in, I'd gained .2 pound, my first gain in months. After this, my weight went up a little and then down a little. I was still compliant with my diet, but my body had reached a new set point. I'd received maximum benefits from this diet. To lose more, I'd have to eat less. I was happy with my new weight. I decided to stick with my plan.

I was now in the dangerous country called "maintenance". The early stages of maintenance are critical. Maintenance is when bad eating habits resurface, and weight is regained. How long is maintenance you ask? Maintenance is forever. I don't mean to frighten you, but you must treat this phase of your diet with the same seriousness as the beginning of the diet. If you can make it through one year of maintenance, relapse is less likely, but still possible.

My body taught me two more lessons. My body is in charge, not my mind or my hopes. I thought I knew what I should weigh, but I didn't. When I switched to a healthy diet, my body decided what my best weight should be. As it turned out, my body's weight choice was lower than mine. My body took me back to college days.

My body also taught me this: Carbohydrate induced cravings are forever. You must deal with it like I've had to. I thought after 14 months, I'd beaten my carbohydrate cravings. Then, I had a bout with a respiratory virus. I decided to drink orange juice for the vitamin C. I knew that orange juice wasn't on my list of foods, but I felt I could cope with the carbohydrates it contained. Wrong! (I hate being wrong so often.) Within 30 minutes, images of ice cream started dancing through my brain. I thought, "I'm sick. Poor me." I bought some ice cream. I did have the presence of mind to buy a small carton. It took only a glass of orange juice mixed with a little self-pity to get my cravings going again. To get back on track, I'd have to go back to what worked in the beginning.

Session 24

My craving dreams returned. This time I dreamed of bread. I wondered why I was dreaming of loaves of bread loaded with butter. As it turned out, I'd added bread to my diet. Gradually, I'd started eating more and more bread. Surprisingly, my weight was stable, but the cravings were a warning sign. As I thought about my history with carbohydrates, I recognized that sweets and candy were not my problem foods. In previous failed diet attempts, I continued to eat flour-based foods like bread and pasta. I now know that baked goods or anything made with flour top my list of problem foods. I don't know why it took me so long to figure this out. When I think of my childhood, the memory of my mother making angel food cake stands out. This was a special event. She whipped 13 eggs by hand, and I watched impatiently until she blended the ingredients and slid the cake into the oven. I remember the smell of the cake as it baked. There are other baked goods memories, but this is the strongest.

I'd also increased the amount of fruit in my diet. Fruits are also a problem food for me. I have no restraint when it comes to fruit. I allow myself to eat a little fruit, but I must limit my fruit intake to berries and apples. I miss fruit more than I miss chocolate. This, too, was a revelation.

Once again, I learned that my impressions about my eating problems and preferences were leading me astray.

Sessions 25 to Present

My body had a few more lessons to teach. Although I'd made it through the holidays without getting back on the carbohydrate wagon, I decided to go to a buffet luncheon which included many dishes which weren't on my diet. After I ate a little of everything and a large piece of cake, I left the table feeling stuffed, sleepy, and miserable. The next day, I hopped on the scale to assess the damage my eating binge had done. My weight was the same, but I felt hungry and my cravings went off the scale. A few days later, I'd gained three pounds. What happened?

Several things happened in my view. First, my experience suggests that our bodies may have metabolic set points. If we eat too much, the body gets rid of the excess. If, however, we eat more food over a sustained time span, the body responds by resetting and putting more energy into fat and pounds.

The body's tendency to compensate for small variations in intake is dangerous in maintenance because our bodies don't punish us immediately for binging by adding pounds. The body waits to see if our food intake change continues. Thus, the body can lull us into thinking we can eat more and still maintain our weight. This is a naughty trick played by the body because it will stack the pounds on a few days later. There is literally "no free lunch."

Like the old saw, "dance with the guy who brought you," the diet which got your weight down is the diet you must stay with. The brain can change its set point, so we have more food cravings. This begins a destructive cycle of eating and weight gain.

My greatest lasting struggle is with night eating. I have persistent cravings after I go to bed. I start thinking about what's in the refrigerator. I know that I should fast for 12 hours to get into ketosis, but my mind won't turn off. I've done better in the last few weeks, but who knows if I'll ever have a night when I don't want to sneak into the kitchen. I didn't think night eating was so important, but it is for me. We decided to track down the literature, and we were surprised to find 217 studies on the subject!

Night Eating: What's It All About?

Night eating isn't just a phenomenon. It's a syndrome. That's right. It's called Night Eating Syndrome or NES. This syndrome was first described in 1955, and NES was recently added to the Diagnostic and Statistical Manual of the American Psychiatric Association. It refers to episodes of binge eating during the night. This disorder is more common among those of us with a high BMI (Olejniczak et al., 2018), those who are genetically sensitive to stress, those who are depressed or for whom food has emotional meaning (Shillito et al., 2018), those who are dependent on nicotine, or those of us who are dissatisfied with our bodies (Stunkard & Lu, 2010). NES may be a unique combination of an eating disorder, sleep disorder, and mood disorder.

Why is NES important? It's important because if you have NES, you'll have more difficulty losing weight (Shillito et al., 2018). Most of us know that we're not supposed to eat late at night if we want to shed unwanted pounds, but we may not know why. Eating during the hours in which the body wants to fast and go into ketosis changes the way we process energy. Energy processing is less efficient.

Night Eating Syndrome is defined by the following:

1. Increased food intake in evening hours and/or at night by consuming at least 25% of total daily consumed food after dinner on at least two nights each week.
2. Three of the following are true:
   a) No desire to eat in the morning or skipping breakfast for four or more mornings each week.
   b) Strong need to eat between dinner and going to bed.
   c) Sleeplessness on four or more nights each week.
   d) Belief one needs to eat to go to sleep or fall back asleep.
   e) Depressive or worsening mood in the evening.
3. Night eating for at least 30 months.
4. Night eating is distressing.

I don't have full blown NES. I meet criteria b and c only. I can control my night eating with will power and a trip to the fridge to grab a pickle. I am finding that I sleep better if I don't raid the refrigerator. Assess yourself honestly. If you meet the diagnostic criteria for NES, read on.

This is what individuals with NES have to say (Shillito et al., 2018).

Maybe it's in my head, I don't know, when you're hungry you know you're hungry. If I want something to eat my belly starts rumbling...
I just feel like I want something...I'm looking for something to make me feel better... so I'll go and get the stuff that does.
Eating always wins you know. I did try on occasions, but I was holding my belly. It was hurtful. My stomach was screaming for food.

Some scientific evidence suggests that NES is linked to changes in brain rhythms and brain chemistry. It is well known that our bodies are governed by rhythms. The most obvious rhythm is our daily rhythm controlling sleep and wakefulness. This rhythm is as regular and as universal as the tides. Our daily rhythms (and we have many) are called circadian rhythms. One study looked at circadian rhythms and transmitter binding in the brain. Serotonin activity in the midbrain is elevated in individuals with NES (Stunkard & Lu, 2010). Remember the importance of serotonin in the food reward system discussed previously. This increased binding of serotonin alters our biological rhythms and our endocrine systems.

Another study found that giving an antidepressant to mice with NES can normalize their eating patterns (Haraguchi et al., 2018). Similar results have been reported when NES patients are given antidepressant medications such as serotonin reuptake inhibitors and Topiramate.

NES, if you have it, requires your serious attention. Discuss your disordered eating pattern with your counselor. If your counselor doesn't know about NES, find a knowledgeable eating disorder treatment center. NES can be treated, and it shouldn't be ignored. If you ignore NES, you may not succeed with your weight loss plan.

The Future

I'd received so many benefits from the ketogenic approach to diet. I decided to summarize these in a Glad List. Read this when you get discouraged to help you keep your eye on the prize.

I continue to go to weekly weigh-ins because I know that they're essential. It's too easy to backslide if one doesn't keep an eagle eye on what one eats. I feel confident that I can maintain this weight. I donated all the clothes which no longer fit. I refuse to hedge my bets. I won't be wearing those clothes again.

About You

We can't predict what your weight loss experience will be. We don't know which lessons you'll learn. What we can tell you is that you'll learn as much as you're open to learning. If you open your mind, allow yourself to take direction from others, and honestly follow a ketogenic diet, you will reap many of the benefits I did. Hopefully, your experiences will energize you to write a better book than this one.

My weight loss center has launched a private website for its clients. It's a safe place where we can share our experiences with the diet, ask and answer questions, and find inspiration when we hit the low spots. I'm going to participate because I know I will continue to need support and sometimes a good talking to if I am to maintain my gains.

MY GLAD LIST

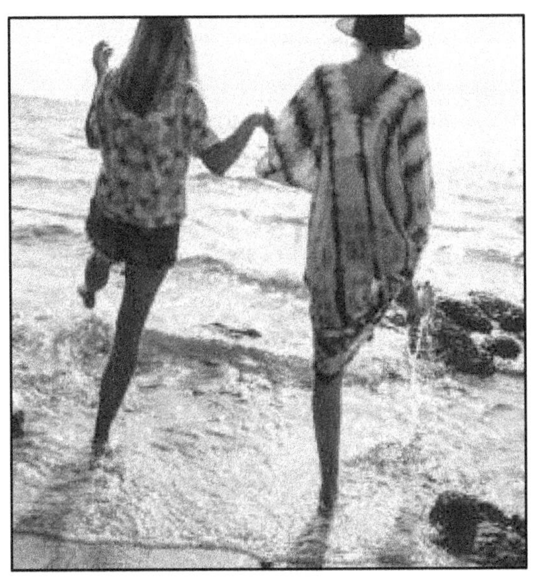

Giving up carbohydrates if you're an addict like me is a daunting exercise. Too many of us give up. I thought it might be helpful to share my Glad List of the benefits of my weight loss program. I borrowed the idea from the movie *Pollyanna*. Whenever, Pollyanna felt blue, she played the Glad Game and thought about something to be glad about. Read my Glad List when you're down, hate yourself because you've relapsed, or think about quitting. These are some of the good things that are waiting for you, the prizes at the end of your weight loss journey. You may not get the same benefits that I did, but you will have your own Glad List if you break your addiction to carbohydrates. Of that, I'm sure. Photo by rawpixel.com from Pexels

- ♥ I'm happier with myself. My self-directed negative thoughts have decreased.
- ♥ My bulging belly is gone.
- ♥ I don't avoid mirrors.
- ♥ I no longer have acid reflux! I'd taken GERD medication for more than 20 years.
- ♥ I don't struggle with constipation (Sorry about the excursion into my bowel function, but it's important to me.)
- ♥ I wear a smaller clothing size. The size I wore in college. I thought that was gone forever.
- ♥ It's easier to do everything from cleaning house to getting into a car.
- ♥ Tight spaces (airplanes, aisles, restaurants, etc.) aren't challenging. I can navigate with ease. No more, excuse me.

- It's fun to move again. I'm not a slug dragging myself about. I feel light and a little like a toddler discovering that his wonderful legs will carry him wherever he wants to go.
- I have more energy. I'm energized by moving. I haven't felt this in years.
- Last and best, I smile more. More people smile and say hello to me. I don't know why, but I feel more connected to the universe.

CHAPTER 18

The diet industry has a deep interest in the failure of dieters—if everyone got skinny, they'd go out of business. —Golda Poretsky

Diet Pills or Appetite Suppressants

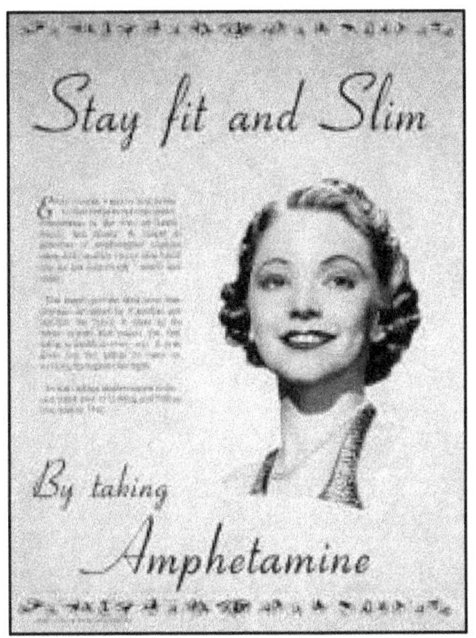

You'd have to be returning from 20 years in a Tibetan monastery to be unaware of the obesity crisis. However, none of us know how to help people lose weight and keep it off. When we funny little monkeys don't know something, we turn to our personal experience or the experiences of those we know. Then we decide, and we stick to our decision no matter what. We might shout out that one and only one type of diet is the sure and certain way to lose weight. Others who've benefitted from weight loss surgery might chime in with, "Surgery is the answer." If we used pills to get the pounds off, we beat the drum for diet pills. The truth is that someone somewhere has lost weight and kept it off using every method ever conceived of by man. With the issue of weight loss, try to keep an open mind. Consider all the options.

We'll state our bias out front. Diet pills scare us. Although we don't like the idea of appetite suppression, appetite suppressants do have their place in a weight loss program. These drugs, however, must be treated with great respect and equal caution.

*** * * ***

In this chapter, we'll tackle two issues—choosing a safe supplement and the utility and safety of appetite suppressants.

Supplement Use and Internet Scams

Most of us take at least one supplement a day. Taking supplements is increasing among both young and older adults. See the chart. Over 40% of our population took supplements in 1988-1994, and over half of us took supplements in 2003-2006 (Gahche, 2011).

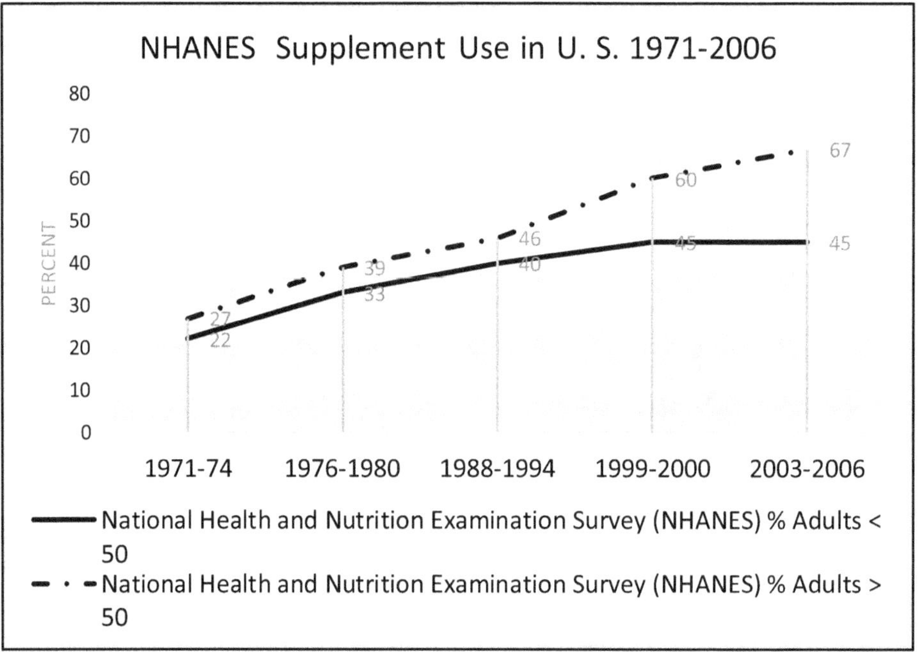

We know that supplements do not undergo rigorous scientific testing and that supplements don't necessarily deliver what they promise. That's old news.

What's new is the recent Federal Trade Commission settlement with Cure Encapsulations. The company made false and unsubstantiated claims for their garcinia cambogia weight loss supplement, and they paid a third-party website to post fake positive reviews on Amazon. The company has agreed to pay a substantial fine. Cure Encapsulations is not alone in their use of a third-party paid review company. Geniux, Alpha Fuel XT, and Spartagen XT are also suspected of this unsavory practice.

Many of us buy supplements on Amazon or other Internet sites, and we rely on customer reviews. This recent action against Cure Encapsulations shows how websites are unable to monitor the claims made by sellers on their sites. The fake review companies are artful and devious.

Since you may find it helpful, as I did, to use supplements during the weight loss process, we'll summarize some ways to determine if a review is fake. This was taken from Rob Miller's blog. https://www.supplementcritique.com/how-to-spot-a-fake-supplement-review-on-amazon/

1. Check out other reviews the supposedly unbiased reviewer has written.
2. Check the dates of the reviews of the product which interests you. A lot of reviews in a single week is suspicious. Honest reviews usually trickle in.
3. Read responses to a criticism of a one-star review. Honest reviewers don't often bother to refute criticisms. Fake reviewers do try to refute criticisms.
4. Fake reviews tend to be short and vague.
5. Look at the distribution of reviews from 1 to 5 stars. Third party companies tend to post a lot of good reviews (five star) and a few bad reviews. Honest reviews will be scattered from one through five. Fake reviewers try to offset a negative review by planting a good one.

Pills That May Make Us Skinny

There are two types of pills which purport to make us skinny—prescription and non-prescription or over the counter (OTC). Prescription pills are developed by pharmaceutical companies and generally undergo some degree of research. We can argue about the quality of the research another time. When you take these products, your usage is monitored by physicians or other health care providers. OTC products may not have any research, and your health care provider may not know you're taking the over the counter product. We'll look at pharmaceutical preparations first.

Pharmaceutical Products

Manufacturers have been busily cranking out all manner of stuff to put in our mouths to make us skinny for the last 70 years. Let's look at stimulants—amphetamine, methamphetamine, Dexedrine, and Benzedrine. These stimulants are the poster children for weight loss drugs. Each of these stimulants acts on the sympathetic nervous system. There are also some illegal stimulants such as cocaine which can curb appetite. The effects of these drugs on weight loss and our brains/bodies are similar. We won't go into the differences among the stimulants. That would require another book.

We're going to go into the history of amphetamine because it was one of the early manufactured drugs used to curb appetite. Amphetamine's history illustrates the hazards of messing about with the biochemistry of the brain.

Amphetamine was first synthesized in 1887 by a Romanian chemist. The drug had no known pharmacological use until 1934 when Smith Kline and French marketed an amphetamine inhaler for nasal congestion. People liked their amphetamine inhalers. The drug made them feel good, gave them energy, kept them awake and alert for hours on end, and stimulated their thinking. By the late 1930s, college students used what they called "pep pills" to increase productivity and allow them to study into the midnight hours.

During World War II, Axis and Allied military commands decided to tap into the stimulating effects of amphetamine and its more potent sister compound, methamphetamine. Pilots taking amphetamines could stay awake longer, and soldiers recklessly charged into battle. It has been reported that 72 million amphetamine tablets were issued during the war.

Did you ever wonder why Kamikaze pilots gave up their lives? It might have been courage, or it might have been the high doses of Pervitin (Japanese amphetamine version) they took before suicide flight missions. The German army ordered front-line soldiers and pilots to take military-issued stimulants which contained a combination of methamphetamine and cocaine.

The dangers of taking amphetamines were evident after the war. In 1945, psychiatrists in military prisons reported large numbers of agitated, hallucinating patients. Many of these patients were behaving bizarrely (e.g., eating their inhalers containing amphetamine).

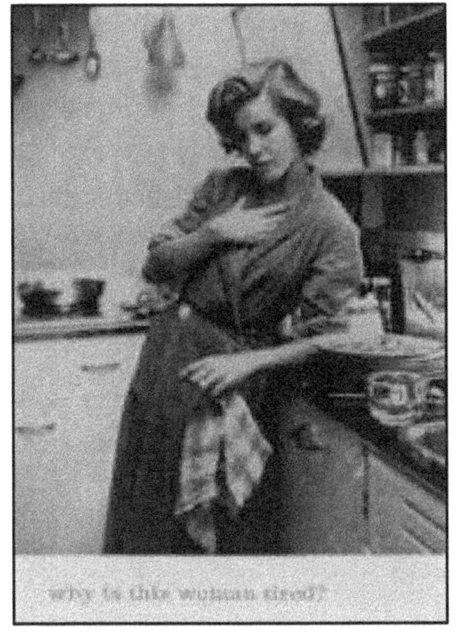

Meanwhile, drug manufacturers were looking for new uses for amphetamines. In 1937, the American Medical Association allowed drug companies to market amphetamine for the treatment of narcolepsy, Parkinson's Disease, mild depression, and hypochondria. In the 1950s, Beatniks took "Bennies" (Benzedrine) to create poetry, music, and art. Amphetamines were also taken by housewives as a "little helper" to get through the monotony of their lives. Women who complained of fatigue were sometimes diagnosed as hypochondriacs and given prescriptions of amphetamine. Long-haul truckers routinely used "speed" so that they could stay on the road longer. In the 1960s, hippies used amphetamines to expand their consciousness.

Stimulants were available without a prescription until 1959 when the FDA began to require prescriptions for Benzedrine. The many harmful effects of stimulants were impossible to ignore. These harmful effects included paranoia, abnormal heartbeat, and heart failure. Despite these side effects, the medical community and the public continued to view amphetamine as harmless. Doctors prescribed amphetamines to vast numbers of their patients. For example, John F. Kennedy received regular injections of methamphetamine mixed with vitamins and hormones from Max Jacobson, nicknamed "Dr. Feelgood." Dr. Jacobson was the doctor to the stars, and he prescribed amphetamines to Cecil De-Mille, Truman Capote, Tennessee Williams, the Rolling Stones, and Congressman Claude Pepper of Florida.

One of the side effects of taking amphetamines for energy was decreased appetite. By the 1960s, amphetamines were prescribed for weight loss. Amphetamine tablets were dispensed by weight loss clinics which often used off-brand products they sold for immense profits (Rasmussen, 2008).

I interviewed many long-term female meth abusers who'd become sober while incarcerated. They all told me that they stayed on meth because the drug made them thin. When they stopped using, they gained weight.

In 1970, the amphetamine epidemic peaked (3.8 million users), and the Comprehensive Drug Abuse Prevention and Control Act established the controlled substance schedules. Only a handful of amphetamine products were placed in Schedule II, meaning many amphetamine products weren't subject to manufacturing quotas or record keeping. Thus, this act did little to curb amphetamine abuse.

The recent amphetamine resurgence began through a combination of recreational drug fashion cycles and an increased illicit supply since the late 1980s. Methamphetamine abuse doubled in the United States between 1983 to 1988. It doubled again between 1988 and 1992, and then quintupled from 1992 to 2002 (Rasmussen, 2008).

Amphetamines and Your Brain

You may think we're wandering a bit here, but there's an important point. Most of us know by now that many stimulant drugs are addictive. When we stop taking them, we experience withdrawal. What many of us don't know is how horribly addictive stimulant drugs can be. We think using these stimulants a few times is harmless. We're wrong. For some vulnerable individuals, only one use of methamphetamine or cocaine is required to alter brain function and produce addiction. Nora Volkow has written extensively on the impact of stimulants on the brain. Her work can be found on the National Institutes of Health website.

Amphetamines produce their stimulating effects by acting on the basal ganglia. How do amphetamines affect the basal ganglia? In the basal ganglia, amphetamines cause brain cells which use dopamine as a transmitter to produce vast amounts of the transmitter. It's this release which makes us feel good. Unfortunately, the brain cannot manufacture dopamine as fast as it is released by amphetamine ingestion. When this happens, the stores of dopamine in the brain are depleted. That doesn't sound too bad, does it? Well, the rub is that stopping the use of these stimulants doesn't make the dopamine manufacturing process return to normal. There is some restoration, but dopamine levels remain low. Depletion of dopamine in the basal ganglia is implicated in the development of Parkinson's Disease.

Thus, there are serious health consequences associated with lowered dopamine levels in the brain which may not show up for years or decades. This long-term impact is associated with the normal decline of dopamine levels in the brain as we age. Thus, stimulant users face the additive effects of aging and depletion of dopamine.

Two case examples illustrate the impact of heavy stimulant use in advanced years, even when abstinence has been achieved. Richard Pryor, a heavy cocaine user, showed prominent Parkinsonian-like tremors and movement problems in his later years. Robin Williams also used stimulant drugs, and he was reported to be developing tremors shortly before he committed suicide.

The important point here is that stimulant drugs which inhibit appetite can cause permanent significant brain damage. Although these effects of amphetamines on the brain were known by the end of World War II, fifty years elapsed before we established the extent and nature of the damage being done. In the interim, millions of people used and abused stimulants. What does this say about over-the-counter diet drugs or newer manufactured drugs which control appetite? Do we understand them any better than doctors and drug companies understood amphetamine and Benzedrine?

Over the Counter Preparations

Over the counter diet drugs can be dangerous. Let's start with the cautionary tale of the man who wore an aluminum foil hat. I evaluated him after he'd been charged with shooting a police officer who'd been called to his home by concerned neighbors. His neighbors were worried because he wandered around his home at all hours, and he'd taken to wearing a homemade aluminum foil hat. When asked about the hat, he stated that aliens were attempting to control his mind. The aluminum blocked their probes. He had barricaded himself in his house because he was afraid, and he shot an officer trying to assist him.

When I first interviewed this man several months after his arrest, he was lucid and pleasant. He no longer feared having his thoughts controlled by aliens. What had happened? Why the drastic change?

When I took his history, this is what I learned. Both he and his wife had weight issues. They tried an herbal preparation marketed in the United States prior to 2004 which contained ephedra, a substance used in traditional Chinese medicine. They were excited about the preparation because it was natural.

They were thrilled when they lost weight, and they started distributing the product and using it regularly over a period of several years.

What they didn't know was that the preparation contained an herb which produces amphetamine-like effects. When ephedra is used for weight loss, it may have tragic side effects including stroke, heart problems, and death. We would add serious mental deterioration to the list. Due to multiple complaints, the FDA stepped in. Ephedra can no longer be advertised as a weight loss preparation. You can still find it in OTC decongestants.

I took an herbal preparation, Phentatrim, to control my appetite. This made me nervous. MRC is supervised by a physician, and they took my health history before suggesting any supplements. I had a health interview with a nurse practitioner. Due to my history of high blood pressure and rapid heart rate, the nurse practitioner recommended Phentatrim rather than a more potent appetite suppressant.

Let's look at what's in Phentatrim. It contains the following active ingredients: Chromium polynicotinate, *Hoodia gordonii* extract, *Lagerstroemia speciosa* extract, and Forskohlil root extract. I didn't know how the herbs acted, so I only took Phentatrim for the first two months. I found I no longer needed appetite suppression after that. I'm happy to report that I had no adverse effects.

What if I'd taken an appetite suppressant I learned about from advertisements? What if I took large doses of one of the Phentatrim ingredients, *Hoodia gordonii*? This appetite suppressant comes from a plant in Africa. It's said that tribesmen in South Africa eat a succulent plant containing *H. gordonii* to reduce appetite and thirst when they're on long treks. Thus far, the mechanisms by which *H. gordonii* acts are unknown. What is known is that some *H. gordonii* products increase blood pressure and pulse rate (Roza, Lovász, Zupkó, Hohmann, & Csupor, 2013).

The cardiovascular effects of *H. gordonii* may be due to sympathomimetic effects (or actions on the sympathetic nervous system). One of these effects is increased thermogenesis (turning on the body's temperature regulation system) which, in turn, may cause weight loss. One reviewer wrote, "Publications based on scientific studies of key aspects such as in vivo biopharmaceutics, the biological activity of the chemical constituents, clinical efficacy, and especially safety are insufficient or completely absent causing great concern as *H. gordonii* is one of the most widely consumed anti-obesity products of natural origin" (Vermaak, Hamman, & Viljoen, 2011).

Many of us like to think that "natural products" are safe. This certainly isn't the case for *H. gordonii*. Had I taken this herb without supervision; I could have had significant medical issues. Many plants are safe at one dose and toxic at another.

The important consideration with any chemical, natural or manmade, which we put in our bodies, is how well it has been studied. For this reason, we cannot recommend any appetite suppressant product. If you decide to use a diet product which suppresses appetite, please, please, please use it according to directions. Don't use any appetite control product for anything other than to jump start your diet process. Use these products under medical supervision by turning to a weight loss program which examines you and your health situation before making herbal recommendations.

More Recent Prescription Weight Loss Products

We can't help but wonder if newer substances which are marketed as appetite control medication also act on the sympathetic nervous system and the brain? Let's look at some of the more recent manufactured products.

Remember the Fen-Phen diet craze of the 1990s? It seemed like everyone we knew was taking Fen-Phen. This drug was represented as a safe approach to appetite suppression which did not cause psychiatric or medical complications. Fen-Phen, the popular name for the combination of fenfluramine and phentermine, was never approved by the FDA for safe use.

Pharmaceutical manufacturers produced the drug to meet the rising demand from clamoring overweight patients around the country. With the popularity of Fen-Phen skyrocketing, American Home Products developed a new version of fenfluramine called dexfenfluramine. This new drug was marketed as Redux and, after intense debate, Redux was approved by the FDA in 1996.

The widespread use of Fen-Phen and Redux was halted when research studies identified alarming side effects of these appetite suppressants. Patients using these appetite suppressants had a 20-fold increase of pulmonary hypertension which is often fatal and a 15-fold increase in heart valve dysfunction (Li et al., 1999).

In response to these findings, the FDA asked the manufacturers of fenfluramine and dexfenfluramine to stop distributing the drugs. Michael Friedman, deputy commissioner of the FDA, issued the following warning: "These findings call for prompt action. The data we have obtained indicate that fenfluramine, and the chemically closely related dexfenfluramine, present an unacceptable risk at this time to the patients who take them." Although the warnings did not include phentermine, the rebuke sent a shock through the drug manufacturing sector, and it was clear that the FDA was closely monitoring activities in this area. For example, in 2010, the stimulant Sibutramine was withdrawn by the FDA due to the increased cardiac risk. Note: You can still take phentermine. It is now called Adipex.

Back to the laboratory for the pharmaceutical manufacturers. In 2012, the FDA approved the first of two new weight loss drugs in over a decade (brand names Belviq/Belviq XR and Qsymia). Since that time, two additional medications have been approved, Contrave and Saxenda. Let's see if these drugs have overcome the problems associated with their predecessors.

Belviq/Belviq XR

Belviq (generic name Lorcaserin), was formulated to be an appetite suppressant which acts on the brain. It is generally recommended for patients with BMIs above 30. It is thought to activate receptors in the brain that allow the neurotransmitter serotonin to be produced and to reduce appetite. Serotonin triggers a feeling of satiety that dampens cravings. Serotonin also is known to influence general mood. According to clinical trials submitted by the manufacturers to the FDA, 50% of dieters who took Belviq were able to lose 5% of their starting weight. On average, this amounted to 12 pounds in one year.

Relatively speaking, this is a small amount of weight loss given the expense, relapse rate, and side-effects involved. Belviq is expensive, and the reported relapse rate exceeded 60%. More importantly, side effects include headaches, dizziness, fatigue, nausea, dry mouth, and constipation. Some patients reported alterations in mood which included depression coupled with agitation.

Qsymia

Qsymia is a combination of the stimulant Phentermine (of Fen-Phen fame) and the anti-seizure drug Topiramate. The trials submitted to the FDA included 3,700 overweight patients. An average weight loss of 9% was recorded for those taking the recommended dosage of Qsymia. That is, on average, patients weighing 200 pounds would have lost approximately 18 pounds during the test trial.

The drug combination in Qsymia is thought to affect weight loss in different ways. Phentermine, of course, is a stimulant that acts to suppress appetite. Topiramate helps you feel fuller and reduces cravings. The most common side effects reported by those taking Qsymia were insomnia, dry mouth, tingling in the extremities, dizziness, and constipation. Less common, but more serious side effects included vision problems and sudden increases in heart rate. Finally, Qsymia can cause mood swings, feelings of depression, and suicidal ideation.

Although there were still some concerns about Phentermine, particularly if overused, the FDA decided the multitude of health problems associated with the exploding obesity epidemic overshadowed the potential side effects of Qsymia.

We have trouble with this logic. Does it make sense to substitute one set of health problems for another, or worse, add a new set of problems to an existing problem?

Contrave

Contrave, approved in 2014, is a combination of two older prescription medications: An antidepressant called bupropion and a drug used to treat addiction called naltrexone. Contrave was initially rejected by the FDA in 2011 due to concerns over cardiovascular risks. It was ultimately approved in 2014.

As with other weight loss drugs, Contrave isn't for those who just want to shed a few pounds or tighten up the abs. This drug is for individuals with a BMI over 30 or obese patients with a related medical condition. Contrave is thought to work on two areas of the brain that regulate both appetite and reward. The dual action of the drugs is said to stimulate central melanocortin pathways which may lead to reduced appetite. Researchers admit that the mechanism by which the combination of drugs induce weight loss is not understood. It is thought that the preparation affects the brain and the way hunger and food are perceived.

In a randomized clinical trial conducted at the Pennington Research Foundation and published in *Lancet*, only 42% of the subjects taking Contrave had a 5% reduction in weight (Greenway et al., 2010). The rest of the subjects didn't lose significant weight.

In addition to the lack of research supporting Contrave's effectiveness, the drug is expensive and comes with a list of worrisome side effects—nausea, headache, constipation, dizziness, dry mouth, blood pressure increases, seizures, and suicidal ideation.

Read what some users said about taking Contrave. Taken from WebMD.

"It was tough for the first month, I had bad nausea. I took some nausea meds to help with that. It's amazing when you get past that. I'm down 30 pounds. I'm not as hungry and don't have cravings, it's a lot easier to eat healthy."

"I took exactly one tablet and I will never take this again! I feel absolutely horrible. I've been on the toilet throwing up and going #2 constantly. I feel sweaty and anxious and disgusting! My entire body feels like it's having a panic attack every 30 min. Do not take it!"

"I discontinued using after six weeks and no weight loss."

"On my third week of Contrave. Noticed a decrease in appetite. I had mild chest pains, extreme nausea as side effects. I am realizing I can't eat much while on the pill or I get extremely nauseated so that's a plus. Haven't lost any weight yet, starting to get discouraged."

"I did not experience any side effects."

Saxenda

Saxenda, approved in 2014, comes with an interesting history in that a lower-dose version, Victosa, has been used to treat Type II Diabetes for many years. This occasionally happens in the unpredictable world of pharmacology. That is, a drug prescribed to treat one illness will produce some side effects related to another illness. In this case, diabetic patients taking Victosa were losing weight.

Unlike other weight loss medications, Saxenda is injected daily. Like other medications, it has been approved for individuals with a BMI greater than 30, or a BMI of 27 with at least one weight-related condition (e.g., high blood pressure). Saxenda (generic name Liraglutide) mimics the hormone GLP-1 which acts to suppress appetite. As well, the drug may assist in normalizing blood sugar.

Clinical trials of Saxenda produced results similar to other medications. That is, in a year-long trial that included 4,800 patients, some received a three-milligram injection, some a placebo. Thirty percent of treated patients experienced a 10% weight loss, while 60% lost 5% or less. Osama Hamdy, MD, Medical Director of the Joslin Diabetic Center commented, "It is not an impressive weight loss for an injectable and expensive medication with lots of potential side effects."

As with the other medications reviewed, common side effects of Saxenda include nausea, vomiting, diarrhea, and constipation. Serious side effects include pancreatitis, gall bladder disease, kidney problems, suicidal thoughts, and increased heart rate.

This is what some users wrote about Saxenda. Taken from WebMD.

"I've tried the drug for a short time and it did not make me feel well. I was dizzy (room spinning). I was so disappointed."

"I started Saxenda since two months and I am on 3 dose almost 2 weeks. I didn't lose any weight at all, even my appetite is still high, only the first week I felt dizzy and tired, but then I believe I developed resistance to the drug. I hope to find related blood test to find out the reason behind such a bad result."

"I've been on medication for 40 days. I have lost 17 pounds and was doing fine until two weeks ago. I started feeling nauseated most of the time. Then I started burping what seemed like an egg taste. After that came vomiting. I cut dose. That worked for about two weeks, so I increased it. The same series of events occurred. It's almost like I ate anything, then later in the day I'll be sick. The stomach pain, vomiting, and diarrhea sent me to the ER yesterday."

"I have been on Saxenda for 1.5 weeks now and have felt nothing, except for the first day I have had no appetite and got a bit burpy. I'm a bit worried that this could be my last hope and it may not work for me. So many people say they lose their appetite and have to force themselves to eat, but still waiting for this 'full feeling'."

What Does All This Mean?

After spending considerable time and energy reviewing research material on weight loss medications, several salient takeaways might help you in your decision-making process. First, solid studies by independent research facilities are lacking for all weight loss products. Most of the studies that have been conducted and reviewed by the FDA were funded and supported by the drug manufacturers in clinical trials. Results of clinical trials, regardless of outcome, are always suspect when the research is funded by the manufacturers of any product.

Second, while the outcome of several studies was positive, it is difficult to sort out the effective intervention. That is, subjects in the studies were encouraged to continue dietary and exercise programs. Which intervention was responsible for the positive outcome—the medication, the diet, or the exercise?

Obviously, better studies are needed. One such study was conducted and reported in the *Archives of Internal Medicine* (Yancy et al., 2010). In this study, subjects were randomly assigned to one of two groups. Subjects in the first group were placed on a low carbohydrate, keto-style diet, while subjects in the second group were placed on the same diet plus a diet pill (Orlistat). After intervention and follow-up, both groups experienced similar weight loss. The keto-only diet was more effective in lowering blood pressure. In other words, the diet pill added little to the treatment outcome. More studies of this nature are needed.

Third, the amount of weight loss reported in these studies does not strike us as significant. Most of the studies reported weight losses between 5%-10%. As noted, patients eligible for weight loss prescription medication are generally required to be obese or overweight (plus one serious medical condition). That would suggest that most patients seeking this intervention would weigh in excess of 200 pounds. A best-case weight loss of 10% would be 20 pounds.

Fourth, and most important, are the troublesome reports of mild to severe side effects. Side effects did not occur in every case, of course, but there is no way to tell in advance which patients would be susceptible to which side effects.

Exercise

Please share any experience you've had with weight loss supplements or diet pills in the forums on our website.
https://www.carbohydrateconfessions.com

CHAPTER 19

Life is uncertain. Eat dessert first. — Ernestine Ulmer

Weight Loss Surgery

I once thought weight loss surgery was too risky or too painful, but I've changed my mind. Weight loss surgery has a place in the treatment spectrum if it is done well and if it is accompanied by support, education, and nutritional counseling.

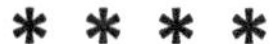

*** * * ***

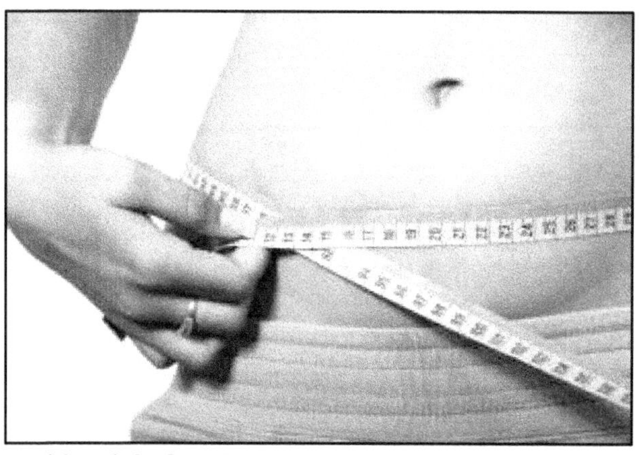

For some of us who've been unable to lose weight by dieting and who have health problems, weight loss surgery can be a viable option. We know people who did benefit from bariatric surgery and some who didn't. The surgical approach to rapid weight loss became popular following its introduction in the mid-1950s. Today, there are more than 250,000 weight loss surgeries performed each year in the United States. Choosing to undergo weight loss surgery is not an easy decision, but for individuals who have struggled with diets, exercise regimens, weight loss pills or supplements, bariatric surgery appears to be the best option when other approaches haven't worked. Photo https://www.pexels.com/photo/woman-girl-fat-fitness-42069/

The most common surgical procedures can be categorized into three basic types: Restrictive surgeries, combined malabsorptive and restrictive, and a miscellaneous procedure category. Restrictive procedures work by shrinking the size of the stomach and slowing down digestion. A normal stomach can hold about three pints of food. After surgery, the restricted stomach may only hold two to three ounces. The logic is simple—the less you eat, the more weight you lose. Vertical sleeve surgery is an example of a restrictive procedure.

Malabsorptive and restrictive surgeries combine reducing stomach size and removing or bypassing a portion of your digestive tract. With a shortened digestive tract, your body absorbs fewer calories. But of course, that means fewer nutrients are absorbed. Surgeons rarely do purely malabsorptive procedures (also called intestinal bypasses) due to their negative side effects. A miscellaneous surgery category includes two new procedures, vBloc Therapy and AspireAssist.

Vertical Sleeve Surgery

In Vertical Sleeve Surgery, a large portion of the stomach is removed, and a new stomach about the size of a banana is created. The new stomach is then attached to the intestines. The smaller stomach makes the patient feel full sooner, and the stomach will secrete fewer hunger-causing hormones. This means lessened hunger after or between meals. Although the volume of the stomach is reduced, rerouting of the intestines isn't done. Nutrient absorption is preserved.

Vertical Sleeve Surgery is done under general anesthesia. The hospital recovery stay is about two days, with full recovery in two to three weeks. This procedure is often recommended for extremely overweight patients because it causes rapid weight loss. The disadvantages of the surgery are risk of infection and the surgery cannot be reversed. Finally, the benefits of the surgery can be negated by overeating (often described as eating through the surgery).

Gastric Bypass Surgery

Gastric bypass is a surgical approach which combines restrictive and malabsorptive elements. Roux-en-Y Gastric Bypass is the most frequently used surgical bypass procedure. In this procedure, the stomach is split into two sections—a small pouch at the top and a larger pouch at the bottom. The intestines are rearranged to connect the top small stomach to a lower section of your small intestines, thus bypassing a portion of the small intestines. The new and smaller stomach causes a sense of fullness, so the patient wants to eat less. Bypassing a portion of the small intestines causes fewer calories and nutrients to be absorbed.

The major advantages of gastric bypass are fast weight loss results and rapid reduction in secondary health risks such as diabetes and cardiovascular complications. Gastric bypass also has good long-term success. Many patients keep the weight they lost off for 10 years or longer.

The disadvantages of gastric bypass include having to follow a strict diet to avoid malnutrition and a dumping syndrome. Dumping syndrome means the food eaten hasn't been fully digested before it enters the small intestines. About 85% of people who receive a gastric bypass experience some symptoms of dumping syndrome. Dumping is triggered by eating high-carbohydrate foods, so adjusting your diet along the lines suggested in this book is essential. Finally, this is an invasive and permanent procedure.

Duodenal Switch

The Duodenal Switch surgery, also known as biliopancreatic with duodenal switch, is the most complex of the weight loss surgeries. The surgery involves both restrictive and malabsorptive procedures. As for vertical sleeve surgery, the restrictive part of the surgery involves removing a large portion of the stomach. The pylorus valve is left intact.

The complex malabsorptive part of the surgery reroutes a lengthy portion of the small intestines. Two pathways are created—one leading from the stomach and the other from the pancreas. These pathways are joined into a common channel just before entering the large intestines. One pathway transports food from the stomach. The other pathway carries bile and digestive juices to the common channel to be mixed with food before it reaches the large intestines. This rerouting reduces the amount of time available to absorb calories from the food in the small intestines.

Weight-loss can be rapid. The patient feels full after eating a smaller amount of food, secretes fewer hunger causing hormones, and absorbs fewer calories. The disadvantages include a longer hospital stay, vitamin and mineral deficiencies, and a strict follow-up diet. Finally, this is an irreversible procedure.

Lap-Band Surgery

In the Lap Band procedure, the stomach isn't altered. Rather, the surgeon places an adjustable band around the upper portion of the stomach. This creates two pouches connected by a very small channel. Emptying of the stomach is slowed.

The lap band surgery has several advantages. The procedure is reversible, it is safer, and patients recover faster. The band can be adjusted in the doctor's office. The major drawbacks are less dramatic weight loss when compared with other surgeries, and weight regain is more likely. Like other procedures, it is necessary to follow a strict diet plan. Most people can eat only a 1/2 to 1 cup of food before feeling full or sick. Food must be soft or well-chewed.

vBloc Therapy

In this procedure, a pacemaker-like device is implanted just below the rib cage adjacent to the vagal nerve. The pacemaker is set to block the action of the vagal nerve. Since the vagal nerve delivers hunger signals from the brain to the stomach, this blocking can reduce appetite. The device is operated by a remote-control device placed outside the body.

Of the weight loss surgeries, vBloc Therapy is the least invasive. The procedure does not require a hospital stay, takes about an hour to complete, and general anesthesia is used. There are fewer complications following this procedure. The disadvantages of the procedure are nausea, vomiting, heartburn, problems swallowing, and chest pain. When the pacemaker battery is drained, a doctor's appointment is necessary to reprogram the device.

Balloon Surgery

In this procedure, a deflated balloon is inserted into the stomach via the mouth. Once the balloon is in place, it is inflated. Weight loss is caused by reducing the amount eaten before a sense of fullness occurs. After six months, the balloon is removed. The average weight loss is reported to be 10%. This procedure is reversible and can be repeated as often as necessary. The major disadvantages are stomachache, nausea, and vomiting. The FDA reported five deaths in 2017 that may have been linked to balloon surgery.

AspireAssist

In this procedure, a tube is inserted into the stomach and then connected to a port on the skin outside the abdomen. After each meal, the patient connects a pump to the port and removes some of the stomach contents.

weight loss occurs because food is removed from the stomach before it can be digested. In a controlled study, patients lost an average of 12% of their total body weight.

The procedure can be completed on an outpatient basis under light anesthesia. The disadvantages are frequent trips to the doctor to adjust the device. A replacement drain tube is required after several uses. The usual side effects include nausea, vomiting, indigestion, constipation, and diarrhea. If the drain tube is removed permanently, the removal can leave an abnormal passageway between the stomach and abdominal wall or fistula.

Dual Dependency

How rude! I've been on a low-carb diet for several months. Now, I'm craving alcohol. What's that about? The problem of dual addiction may not seem relevant to bariatric surgery and weight loss, but it is. Stick with us.

Backstory: Years ago, my husband and I had a gin and tonic before dinner. Eventually, it became two, then three gin and tonics. What worried me was the gin clock ticking away in my brain. I knew when it was four o'clock because I became very, very thirsty. I could see the lovely gin and tonic waiting for me at home. My thirst increased steadily during the drive home. When I started the diet program, I was drinking no more than one or two drinks per month.

Most diet programs suggest cutting back or eliminating alcohol from your diet. Cutting back on alcoholic beverage consumption is particularly important in a low carb diet program because all alcoholic beverages contain carbohydrates. Most mixed drinks are loaded with sugar. When I started my diet, I wasn't worried about this requirement because I hadn't overused alcohol for years.

Approximately three months into the diet, I began craving a gin and tonic about four PM. Does that sound familiar? I asked myself, "Did reducing food-based carbohydrates rekindle my dormant alcohol abuse pattern?" Since both food and alcohol are addictive, does having one addiction make you vulnerable to another? Scientists call having more than one addiction a co-morbidity. People like me who are addicted to cigarettes, alcohol, and carbohydrates have co-morbid addictions with an increased relapse rate.

We were surprised to learn that cutting back on carbs could cause many people to drink more alcohol. Some increased their alcohol consumption to the point that they had diagnosable alcohol abuse. The upturn in alcohol abuse diagnoses in people who underwent bariatric surgery also surprised surgeons.

In fact, many surgeons denied the possibility of an uptick in substance abuse incidence after bariatric surgery. The evidence that bariatric surgery can cause a substance dependence has piled so high that surgeons are now looking for ways to address this complication.

After gastric bypass surgery, patients with no prior history of alcohol abuse started drinking more alcohol. The new drinkers hadn't consumed alcohol to excess before surgery (Chang et al., 2018). While the problem drinking was not immediately apparent in post-surgical follow up, patients began reporting problem drinking after a delay—six months to two years after surgery (Blackburn, Hajnal, & Leggio, 2017; DuBreuil, 2017). The patients' alcohol consumption was not a casual beer with a buddy. These folks had become problem drinkers with diagnosed substance abuse disorders.

What about gastric banding surgery? Does having a gastric banding procedure increase problem drinking? Thus far, it appears that gastric banding does not produce delayed problem drinking. This finding, if replicated, suggests that increased alcohol consumption is not related to getting fewer rewarding goodies into the digestive system. Both procedures reduce the amount of food eaten. The stomach holds less after both procedures.

The increased problem drinking after gastric bypass got animal researchers' attention, and they developed animal models of bariatric surgery. They looked at the effect of bariatric surgery in mice who were addicted to a high-fat diet. Mice were fed a high-fat diet, and then the bariatric surgery was performed. Would mice increase their consumption of ethanol (100% pure alcohol) after the surgery? Would mice work to gain access to alcohol? The answer to both questions was "yes". Mice drank more alcohol after surgery, and they worked to obtain it (Gregorio et al., 2016). Mice and men that are addicted to fat drink more alcohol after bariatric surgery.

How do we explain this? Ochner and colleagues discussed the complexity of the relationship between substances released from the gut (peptides) and the brain (Ochner et al., 2012). They suggest that there may be persistent reward-related mechanisms in the limbic system which drive food intake. This drive to consume continues even though our behavior, our stomach size, and our food intake change.

Why is this important to the recovering carbohydrate addict? If you are considering a gastric bypass procedure, you must discuss the risk of increased alcohol consumption with your health care provider. There may be a lower risk of alcohol abuse after gastric banding, but caution is warranted. If you don't plan to undergo a weight loss procedure, caution is still warranted. Losing weight does not guarantee that the brain mechanisms linked to your other addictions have completely recovered. These old addictions could pop back into your life like a meddlesome relative.

Summary

The more weight you need to lose the greater is your need for medical supervision and serious consideration of bariatric surgery. You can't become a candidate for bariatric surgery unless you meet the criteria of the medical facility of your choice. For example, most surgeons won't accept patients with a BMI less than 30. Occasionally, patients in the 25–30 BMI range are accepted for surgical treatment if serious medical complications are linked to the weight status, or the individual has tried multiple interventions in the past. Weight-loss surgery is viewed by the medical establishment as a serious intervention of last resort.

No matter how you slice it (no pun intended), you're going to have to change the way you eat to get back to a healthy weight. If you undergo surgery and you don't change the way you eat, you'll get the weight back.

Not all surgery programs are created equal. Choose carefully. Look for a surgeon with a support program offering regular visits with dietitians and support staff as well as strong success rates. We recommend supplementing bariatric surgery with enrollment in a low carbohydrate weight loss program.

Questions You Might Ask

If you're thinking about bariatric surgery, you might ask the following questions.

- What percentage of patients drop out after surgery and why do they drop out?
- What percentage of patients achieve a healthy weight after the proposed surgery?
- What is the risk of complications with the procedure and what percentage of patients have these complications?
- What are the long–term mechanical complications associated with the bariatric surgery?
- What is the risk for malnutrition after bariatric surgery and how is it managed?

- What is the extent of disease remission (e.g., Type II Diabetes) with bariatric surgery?
- Will this bariatric surgery improve your long-term health?

Exercise

Have you accepted that all weight loss options require a long-term change in diet and eating pattern?

CHAPTER 20

*Old age is not so bad when you consider the alternatives. —
Maurice Chevalier*

I Can't Lose Weight. I'm Too Old

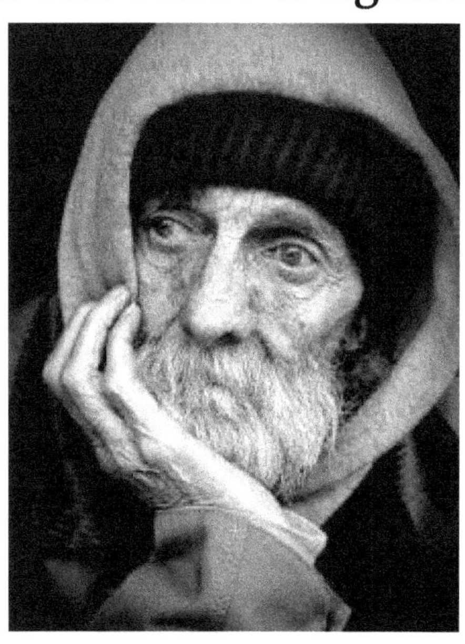

The main reason I'd lived with my extra pounds for as long as I did was my age. I'm a senior lady, and I thought the reason I couldn't drop the pounds like I once did was my age. When I complained to my doctors that I couldn't get the pounds off, more than one agreed that I just might have to live with the extra pounds. Well, don't you believe the myth that old folks can't lose weight.
Photo
https://www.pexels.com/photo/man-person-people-old-34534/

* * * *

It will come as no surprise that older adults are getting fat too. Currently 20% of adults 65 years or older are classified as obese. This percentage will increase as the baby boomers become seniors (Villareal et al., 2011).

Although being an overweight senior is common, there is little information to guide physicians, let alone we lay folks, on what to do about being overweight and a senior. Some care providers worry that the stress of losing weight may be more dangerous than continuing to be overweight. Some also suggest that it's harder for seniors to lose weight because old folks have a lifetime of bad eating habits. Boy! The last sentence makes me burn—a medical version of you can't teach an old dog new tricks. Some health providers are concerned that losing weight past the age of 65 will cause the dieter to lose lean muscle and bone mass (Beavers et al., 2014). All these concerns are perceptions based on no evidence.

Villareal and colleagues did a pioneering study in 2011. They followed 93 people who were over 65 and overweight. The subjects were enrolled in one of four groups—diet group, exercise group, diet plus exercise, and control (continue with usual diet and exercise). Quality of life, physical performance, and body composition were measured before and after treatment. Diet, exercise, or a combination of the two made people stronger and were beneficial. The combination of diet and exercise provided the most benefits.

Waters followed 16 seniors for 30 months on weight loss and physical activity interventions (Waters, 2013). The older adults maintained both their weight loss across the 30 months of the study and had clinically significant improvements in physical function and insulin sensitivity. The authors concluded, "Thus, long-term intentional weight loss and fat loss appears possible in obese, older adults."

Beavers et al. followed up on Waters' study by asking ambulatory overweight or obese seniors between the ages of 60 to 79 to participate in a long-term study of weight loss and exercise. They looked at cardiovascular risk factors, mobility, and body composition. An 18-month behavioral weight loss and mobility program was successful in achieving and maintaining stable weight loss in most subjects. Two-thirds of the weight loss was from fat mass. The lean mass percentage of the subjects was increased. More importantly, cardiovascular and metabolic disease risk factors as well as mobility were improved.

The authors stated, "Strength and power can be maintained during weight loss even by seniors and attenuation of lean muscle mass loss in older adults is prudent and is currently recommended."

Villareal and colleagues wanted to compare the relative health benefits of either aerobic or resistance exercise when combined with a weight loss diet (Villareal et al., 2017). They recruited 160 overweight adults and assigned them to one of the following treatment groups: Weight loss only, weight loss plus aerobic and resistance exercise, weight loss plus aerobic exercise, and weight loss plus resistance exercise. The researchers measured changes in physical performance, frailty, body composition, and mineral bone density. The results showed that subjects following a weight loss program and doing both aerobic and resistance exercise improved more than subjects in the other groups.

It's not too late to teach old dogs new tricks! In fact, evidence is accumulating that older adults can lose and maintain weight loss better than younger adults (Nguyen et al., 2008). When it comes to weight loss maintenance, it's easier to teach an old dog than a young one.

Bottom Line

You can't use your age as an excuse to avoid tackling your weight issues. You can lose weight at any age. Losing weight in your senior years confers health and quality of life benefits. As always, consider your individual health situation, and don't go crazy. See a doctor and set reasonable goals.

CHAPTER 21

*Old age is when broadness of the mind and narrowness of the
waist change places. — Red Skelton*

Old, Happy, and Healthy

Now that we've hopefully convinced you that it's never too late to get the
pounds off, let's look at some other goodies which impact health, weight,
and longevity.

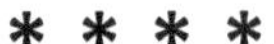

*** * * ***

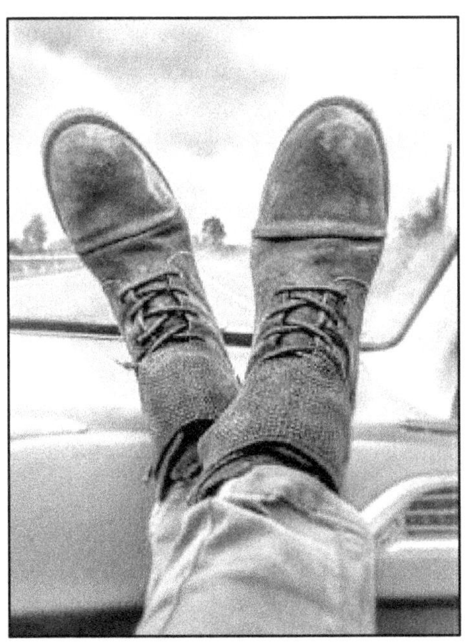

When Do You Become Old?

Are you old when you reach 40, 50, or 60? The multifaceted MURDOCK project found that physical decline begins early in the life cycle. That is, people don't suddenly "get old" at some preset age. Rather, physical change is a long-term process. The human body is made up of fat, lean tissue (muscle/organs), bones, and water. After age 30, people tend to gradually lose lean tissue. Through atrophy, your muscles and organs may lose some of their cells. Bones may become less dense, and tissue loss may reduce the amount of water in your body. These body changes with aging show up in our height. How tall were you at age 18? How tall are you now? We typically lose about one-half inch every 10 years after age 40. Height loss is even more rapid after age 70. Photo by Juan Antonio Fatuarte León from Pexels

The researchers at the Murdock project suggest that many of the effects of aging can be slowed by following a healthy diet, staying active, maintaining positive social relationships, finding a purpose in life, and laughing a lot (Henderson, 2018). Hey! Maybe if you're not getting shorter at the expected rate, you're doing a good job of taking care of your health.

How Did I Grow that Belly Fat?

A recent Mayo Clinic report described the tendency to gain weight during middle age and to accumulate weight in the belly region (Kapoor, Collazo-Clavell, & Faubion, 2017). This central fat distribution is common among women in midlife. We don't know where the belly fat came from. The fat accumulation may be due to aging, decreased estrogen levels after menopause, genetic makeup, or not following a healthy lifestyle.

Men don't have the same tendency to develop an apple belly. Why? No one knows. Maybe it's the differences between our sex hormones and the way they shift during middle life. Maybe it's because men and women have different cravings, and we react to our cravings uniquely. In a study of 1,000 Americans, women's comfort foods are ice cream, cookies, and chocolate. Men prefer hearty warm foods such as pasta or steak. When women eat their favorite comfort foods, they feel guilty. When men eat comfort foods, they don't feel one bit guilty (Wansink, Cheney, & Chan, 2003). Guilt makes cortisol and cortisol makes fat. Do women's guilt and shame give them an apple belly?

Although this suggestion falls in the not fun category, let's see if your apple belly is something to worry about. Let's measure it. Stand and place a tape measure around your bare stomach, just above the hip bone. Make sure the tape is level all the way around and snug against your skin. Relax, exhale and measure, resisting the urge to suck in your stomach. For women, a measurement of more than 35 inches indicates the accumulation of excess visceral fat which can contribute to health problems. For men, a waist measurement of more than 40 inches signals a similar cause for concern.

Back to Exercise

Although we don't have to exercise to lose weight, exercise plus dieting may have extra health benefits for seniors. Remember the Villareal study (Villareal et al., 2017)? After one year of weight loss plus exercise (aerobic and resistance), physical performance, oxygen consumption, bone mineral density, balance, and gait improved. The subjects lost 10% of their body weight in the combined weight loss exercise group. It's important to note that exercise alone was not helpful with weight loss. This result is consistent with previously cited studies involving younger subjects.

In summary, we seniors don't have to be jocks, but a combination of a light exercise and weight loss as low as 10% can bring immense benefits. Done carefully, exercise and diet are likely to cause no serious injuries or ill-effects. The Mayo Clinic recommends 30 minutes of moderate aerobic exercises each day and mild weight training twice a week. The moderate aerobic exercise can include a brisk walk, bicycling in the park, water aerobics, or rebounding. Most dietitians recommend consuming a protein supplement one to two hours after an active workout.

In her book *Fit Over Forty*, Sherri MacMillan recommends modest weight training. As you get stronger, gradually increase your weight load (MacMillan, 2001). She cautions, "Don't rush it. Progress no more than 5-10 percent every two weeks to minimize strain on your tendons, ligaments, and muscles."

Longevity Diet

Two health-related projects provide helpful information on longevity. Valtor Longo, a biochemist and head of the Longevity Institute of the USC School of Gerontology, has devoted decades to understanding the connections between nutrition and healthy aging. Stemming from a variety of studies on successful aging, Dr. Longo developed the Longevity Diet (Longo, 2018).

The Longevity Diet is similar to the ketogenic diet, and there's solid science behind it. The Longevity Diet recommends the following:

- Eat vegetables of all sorts.
- Eat 2 to 3 servings of good fish high in Omega 3 fatty acids per week.
- Limit the amount of red and white organic meats.
- Eat eggs.
- Eat a moderate amount of beans and peas.
- Eat nuts and olive oil high in Omega 3.

- Don't eat for four hours before bedtime.
- Confine food intake to a 12-hour period.
- Fast during the remaining 12 hours.

Longevity Hotspots Around the Globe

There are places scattered about our globe where most folks live into their 90s and beyond. Daniel Buettner calls these Blue Zones. Mr. Buettner, a *National Geographic* explorer and journalist, went on a quest in 2000 to find the lifestyle secrets of longevity in five regions across Europe, Latin America, Asia, and the United States. These regions were previously identified by researchers as having the highest concentration of people who lived past age 100. Not only did seniors in these regions live past 100, but they were relatively free of Western diseases.

The following regions were given Blue Zone status: Ikaria, Greece; Okinawa, Japan; Ogliastra, Sardinia; Nicoya, Costa Rica; and Loma Linda, California. In 2004, Buettner rounded up a team of anthropologists, demographers, and epidemiologists. The team traveled to the five regions to study elderly subjects for several months. The researchers observed the habits and customs of the seniors, conducted group meetings, and interviewed individuals. The project's goal was to determine if these regions had any health habits in common.

Buettner and his team wrote several fascinating books. However, for our purposes, we'll focus on the lessons for living longer from the people who've lived the longest. These lessons are summarized in Buettner's first book, *The Blue Zones* (Buettner, 2008). We divided the lessons into six major categories.

Exercise

People in the Blue Zones do some modest physical activity each day. They take advantage of small inconveniences such as parking some distance from a storefront, taking stairs rather than elevators, and riding a bike rather than driving a car.

Food Habits

People in the Blue Zones don't rush through their meals. They eat at a table and with friends and family. They don't eat in front of the television or while driving. Enjoy each bite. Mindless eating makes you fat.

People in the Blue Zones stop eating before they feel full. Fullness may be difficult for the novice to estimate, but with practice, people are able to stop just short of the stuffed feeling. Or, as one doctor put it, "Eat so you are no longer hungry, but not full."

Veggies, Veggies, Veggies

Across the diverse Blue Zones, there was a general preference for plant-based foods. Fresh fruits and vegetables are included in all meals. Meat is generally discouraged, with small portions consumed two or three times a week.

Alcohol

People in the Blue Zones neither abstain from alcohol nor drink to excess. Many seniors in the Blue Zones sip a glass of wine each day with a friend. Dark red wine is recommended.

A Purpose to Life

Most of the elderly people in the Blue Zones do something which gives them a sense of purpose and challenges them. These include board games, formal classes, or learning some new skill (e.g., learning an instrument, a new language, or a computer game).

People in the Blue Zones are thankful for each day. They define their intention or purpose each day. Read R. E.'s intention.

Dear Creator: My deepest thanks for granting another day to enjoy the blessings and gifts of this wondrous earth. Surely, today I am fortunate to be alive, to have precious human life, grant me the strength not to waste it. I will use all my energies to develop myself, to expand my heart out to others, to achieve enlightenment for the benefit of all beings. I thank you for the opportunity to care for my dear family. Let me go forth with an intention to benefit my fellow beings by my actions, words, and thoughts. I am going to have kind and compassionate thoughts for others, I am not going to get angry or think badly of others. Give me the strength to carry out your design and actualize your intent for me. Going forward into this day, may I benefit all beings I encounter. May I live moment to moment in accepting awareness.

Relax and Savor

Centenarians in the Blue Zones exuded a sense of serenity. They have learned that precious moments pass us by if we blindly lurch toward some fleeting material goal. Instead, they advised us to treasure the precious moments. Watch a small animal play, listen to the laughter of children, smell the aroma of a bouquet, enjoy a colorful sunset, relax to some beautiful music, or caress a loved one.

Enjoying small but precious moments during a day can help reduce stress, which in turn can reduce inflammation. Enjoying precious moments, along with prayer, contemplation, or meditation, can help slow down the incessant and disturbing internal chattering of the mind.

Summary

The myth of old age is mostly a concoction of economic mismanagement and cruel politics. Old age is often thought of as the arbitrary and ill-defined age of retirement, which for most seniors is 65 years old. Studies reviewed in this chapter suggest that aging begins shortly after age 30 and continues at a steady pace.

We can find peace and joy in precious moments. Life is short—don't miss it!

CHAPTER 22

If you ask what is the single most important key to longevity, I would have to say it is avoiding worry, stress, and tension. And if you didn't ask me, I'd still have to say it. — George Burns

Ketogenic Diet: A Fountain of Youth?

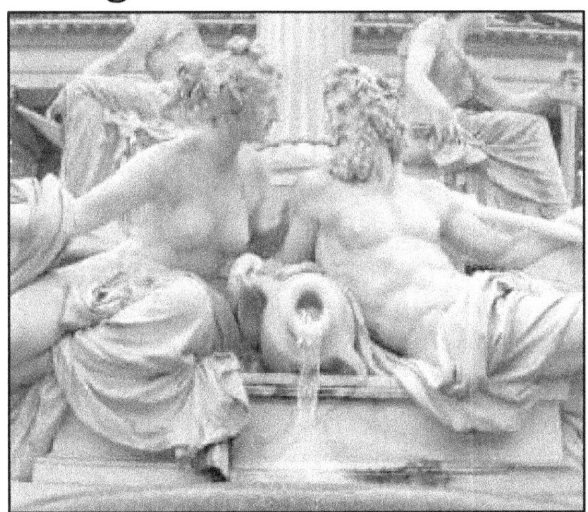

Throughout this offering, I've railed and ranted. Now, it's time for the ranting to end and the cheering to begin. I started a ketogenic diet because I wanted to lose weight. That was my only goal, to get rid of Caroline, my belly fat. The possible health benefits of the diet, other than the indirect effects of weighing less, didn't occur to me. Image by <a href="https://pixabay.com/users/jensjunge-402508/

As my curiosity about the major impact this diet was having on my emotions as well as my weight developed, I began to read, to study the ketogenic diet. What I found surprised and amazed me. Not only are ketogenic diets good for weight loss, but they promise enormous benefits for our health and well-being. Although the research on the health benefits of a ketogenic lifestyle is in its infancy, the promises that following a ketogenic diet will reduce the impact of illness and improve our quality of life as well as our longevity are there.

I must thank the many researchers who have gone against the grain and studied the impact of the ketogenic diet. I think future scientists will regard them as prescient leaders of a quiet revolution.

* * * *

Toward a Definition of the Ketogenic Diet

Not all ketogenic diets are equivalent. The diet you follow may not be the diet used by your friend down the street (Veyrat-Durebex et al., 2018). In general, the term ketogenic diet refers to a high-fat, low-carbohydrate, and adequate-protein diet (Zhang, Xu, Zhang, Yang, & Li, 2018). Most ketogenic diets limit carbohydrates to 20 to 30 grams per day or less than 5% of total daily calories (Bosco et al., 2018). To make up for the energy deficit caused by reduced carbohydrate intake, fatty foods are added to the diet. When this low carbohydrate state is maintained for more than 45 days, the liver begins to produce ketone bodies from fatty acids by a process called ketosis.

The most important medical application of the ketogenic diet is the control of epileptic seizures (Lefevre & Aronson, 2000). Using diet to control epileptic seizures dates to the fifth century A.D. when it was thought that fasting helped control epileptic seizures. In the 1920s, pediatricians at Johns Hopkins Medical Center examined this notion and found that starvation did impact seizure frequency, and they discovered that the antiepileptic effect came from ketosis, or the presence of ketone bodies in the circulation. These doctors demonstrated that it wasn't necessary to starve oneself to achieve the state of ketosis. This state happens when we limit the intake of carbohydrates and force our bodies to switch from using carbohydrates as our energy source to using fat.

Ketosis must not be confused with diabetic ketoacidosis. Diabetic ketoacidosis is a complication of diabetes mellitus that results in too little insulin in the body. The level of ketones and sugar in the blood go to dangerously high levels and, as a result, blood acidity rises. Diabetic ketoacidosis is life threatening and can damage internal organs like the liver and kidneys.

Benign ketosis, on the other hand, is a controlled insulin regulated process which results in a mild release of fatty acids and ketone body production.

The classic ketogenic diet, developed at Johns Hopkins, recommended fats in a 4:1 ratio to carbohydrates. These fats come from long-chain fatty acid foods such as oils (olive and soybean), fish, nuts, avocado, and meat. Fatty acids are the basic building blocks of lipids or fats. They are classified by the number of carbon atoms in their tails. Those with 14 or more carbon atoms are long-chain fatty acids.

For research purposes, the most widely used ketogenic diet is the Modified Atkins Diet or MAD (Kossoff & Dorward, 2008). The classic 4:1 ketogenic diet is difficult for many of us to tolerate. The MAD was developed to address this concern. The MAD is well accepted by patients and compliance with this diet is superior to a low-fat diet.

The lack of a precise definition of a ketogenic diet makes it difficult to assess the research on the possible health benefits of each diet. In research studies, carbohydrate consumption may be as low as 4% or as high as 40% of daily caloric intake (Iacovides & Meiring, 2018). Since researchers are using different protocols, the research findings summarized here should be viewed with this limitation in mind.

How Does Ketosis Help Us Lose Weight?

Atkins's original hypothesis suggested that weight loss on his low carbohydrate diet was induced by losing energy through excretion of ketone bodies. Since Atkins, other hypotheses have been proposed to explain the rapid weight loss that is often found when compared to low-calorie or low-fat diets. The exact mechanism or mechanisms by which the ketogenic diet produces weight loss is, as yet, unknown. Several theories have been advanced.

1. Ketosis is a more efficient process. The use of energy from protein and fat in a ketogenic diet is an inexpensive process for the body. It takes more metabolic fuel to convert glucose to energy than it does to convert proteins and fats. There is little evidence to support this notion (Paoli, 2014).

2. We're less hungry when we don't eat carbohydrates. Some argue that low carbohydrate diets reduce our appetites and appetite control hormones due to the actions of the ketone bodies.

3. Fewer fat cells are produced and more are broken down.

4. The body's respiratory quotient is reduced on a ketogenic diet.

Are Ketogenic Diets Dangerous?

When I told a close friend I was using a low carbohydrate diet to lose my unwanted pounds, her forehead furrowed, and a look of concern crept across her face. She was worried that I was jeopardizing my health by cutting back carbohydrates and increasing fats. She is not alone in this concern. We regular folks and medical professionals worry about the safety of a ketogenic diet. Let's put those worries to rest right now. Castro et al. said it best, "... there is still some distrust regarding the very low carbohydrate ketogenic diet despite solid scientific evidence that supports the use of this kind of diet as useful in weight loss therapy" (Castro et al., 2018).

Paoli et al. studied individuals between the ages of 25 to 65 years of age who followed what they described as a ketogenic Mediterranean diet enhanced with phyto extracts (Paoli, Bianco, Grimaldi, Lodi, & Bosco, 2013). Most of the subjects lost significant weight and body fat, and they maintained their weight losses. Better yet, subjects who started a ketogenic diet stayed on it. Sticking with a diet is a major problem for us all. We stay with a ketogenic diet for two reasons. First, it works. Second, we feel good while losing weight.

Anyone working with weight loss can tell you that the major barrier to sticking with a diet is hunger and the associated miseries of cutting back on calories (Castro et al., 2018). Your body hates this, and it tells you so in no uncertain terms. Within a few days to a week, we are hungry, irritable, and depressed. Staying with a ketogenic diet is easier. Many of us have a period of lethargy in the first week or two on the diet. In the lay literature, this is called the keto flu. The flu-like symptoms happen because our bodies are shifting gears from carbohydrates to fat. The universal positive experience most of us get almost immediately is not feeling hungry. Scientists don't know why this is, but some believe that ketosis has an anorexigenic effect. In lay terms, this means that the diet makes us disinterested in food.

Health care providers have voiced a number of concerns about the ketogenic diet (Bosco et al., 2018). The primary worry of these health care providers is the issue of high cholesterol. Will eating additional fat increase the lipids in our blood? Will the diet cause a rise in LDL cholesterol and triglycerides? This concern, however, appears to be unwarranted. Several lines of evidence show that following a ketogenic diet has a beneficial impact on cardiovascular risk factors. These benefits include reduced total cholesterol, decreased levels of glucose in the blood, increased HDL, reduced blood triglycerides, and increased size and volume of LDL–C particles (Paoli, 2014). In addition, reducing dietary carbohydrates can lead to inhibition of cholesterol production.

Will following a ketogenic diet also benefit those of us with the metabolic syndrome? When insulin resistance develops as part of the metabolic syndrome, the muscle cells don't take up circulating glucose. A greater proportion of the carbohydrates eaten are converted to fat rather than being used for energy. Following a ketogenic diet improves glycemic control.

Another common sticking point for health care providers is the safety of long-term adherence to a ketogenic diet. Will organs such as the kidneys be damaged as they struggle to get rid of the excess ketones? In Paoli's study, ketogenic diets didn't change kidney function (ALT, AST, creatinine or BUN). There is a high level of nitrogen excretion during protein metabolism, and this could increase pressure on the kidneys. Elevated kidney markers are not a problem for healthy people; however, individuals with renal insufficiency may be more susceptible to these effects. For these individuals, medical supervision during the diet process is essential.

Some have worried that following a ketogenic diet will affect muscle strength and lead to loss of muscle mass. Will the diet make us weak? Will we lose muscle rather than fat? Castro et al. followed dieters on a ketogenic diet for one to two years. The muscle mass and strength of the dieters were maintained. The weight loss these dieters experienced was due to reduced fat mass not reduced muscle mass. Vargas et al. studied men undergoing resistance training while on a ketogenic diet. They found decreased fat mass and decreased abdominal or visceral fat. Lean body mass was not decreased (Vargas et al., 2018). Male artistic gymnasts used a ketogenic diet for 12 weeks. They lost weight, but they did not lose muscle strength or muscle mass (Kephart et al., 2018). Bodybuilders on a ketogenic diet gained muscle mass and strength at the same rate while losing body fat. Finally, a sample of clients at a CrossFit facility tried the ketogenic diet for 12 weeks (low carbohydrate, moderate protein, high fat). Muscle mass was maintained during resistance training, but fat mass was reduced. They concluded that the program did not "compromise weightlifting, running, or aerobic performance" (Kephart et al., 2018).

Some are troubled by the possibility that following a ketogenic diet will starve the brain. After all, the brain uses glucose as its primary energy source. What happens when you force the brain to use ketones as an energy source?

The ketone bodies produced by the liver when you reduce the amount of carbohydrates you consume can be used for energy by the brain (Fan, 2013). The three major ketone bodies are beta-hydroxybutyrate, acetoacetate, and acetone. The liver produces ketone bodies derived from the fatty acids in your body fat or diet. These ketones are released into the bloodstream and are taken up by the brain. In the brain, the mitochondria, sometimes called energy factories, can metabolize ketone bodies.

Not only can the brain use ketone bodies as an energy source, but there are probable benefits to using ketones rather than glucose as an energy source. Ketones may be protective against an array of brain diseases. Despite their superficial differences, many neurological diseases share one major problem—deficient energy production. Ketones can help solve this problem by serving as an alternative energy source. One of the ketone bodies, beta-hydroxybutyrate, may be a more efficient source of energy than glucose. Also, the ketogenic diet increases the number of mitochondria in the brain.

Ketone bodies may also protect the brain from the neuronal stress caused by cellular metabolism. The reactive oxidants produced by cellular metabolism bombard proteins and membranes wrecking their structure. Increased oxidants are linked to aging, stroke, and neurodegeneration. In addition, low carbohydrate consumption reduces the glucose oxidation which stresses mitochondria.

Castro et al. (2018) studied neurocognitive processes such as learning, attention, decision making, and memory as well as the quality of life of individuals on a ketogenic diet. The thought processes of individuals on the ketogenic diet were improved. The patients on the diet lost weight, but they had increased physical activity, better sleep, improved sexual function, decreased food cravings, and an improved sense of well-being. Difficulty sleeping, lethargy, decreased libido, and depression are all linked to being overweight. In a study of 18 children with treatment resistant epilepsy placed on a ketogenic diet, the children had an increased total sleep, better slow wave sleep, increased rapid eye movement sleep, and a decrease in sleep stage II (Bostock, Kirkby, & Taylor, 2017).

Some have worried that the diet may not show negative effects in the short-term, but what about the long-term? Long term data is always hard to find for any health intervention. What we did find suggested that a ketogenic diet can be maintained without major health problems for several years (Heussinger et al., 2018).

Ketogenic Diet and Cancer

Ketogenic diets are gaining traction as adjuvant or supportive treatments for several types of cancer (Ok et al., 2018). Some physicians are reluctant to use a ketogenic diet with cancer patients despite evidence of its utility (Cohen, Fontaine, Arend, Soleymani, & Gower, 2018). The ketogenic diet does not replace other treatments, but it is used as a supplement. The ketogenic diet targets the Warburg effect. The Warburg effect is a biochemical phenomenon in which the distinctive metabolic properties of cancer cells are targeted to slow their growth or destroy them. Cancer cells rely on glycolosis or the breakdown of glucose to obtain energy to survive and grow. Many cancer cells cannot use ketone bodies as an energy source due to a mitochondrial dysfunction and the lack of the enzymes necessary to use ketone bodies as fuel. The rationale for providing a fat-rich, low-carbohydrate diet in cancer therapy is to reduce circulating glucose levels and induce ketosis. The cancer cells are starved while the normal cells adapt their metabolism, use the available ketone bodies, and survive (Weber, Aminazdeh-Gohari, & Kofler, 2018). The restricted access to glucose during a ketogenic diet increases oxidative stress in cancer cells. Also, reducing blood glucose reduces insulin growth factors which drive cancer cell proliferation. As a result, the rate of cancer cell growth is inhibited under low blood glucose conditions.

Glioblastoma

McGill-Martin et al. described the use of a ketogenic diet as an adjuvant therapy with glioblastoma patients as "gathering momentum" (Martin-McGill, Marson, Tudur Smith, & Jenkinson, 2018). The ketogenic diet is tolerated, has limited side effects, and is attractive to patients. Of the several types of brain cancer, glioblastoma has a very poor survival rate. A glioblastoma is a brain cancer involving the glial cells of the brain. Glia are cells which support the nerve cells of the brain.

Santos et al. used a ketogenic diet to induce hypoglycemia in patients with high grade glioblastomas (Santos et al., 2018). They also used a standard diet as a comparison. The response rate of patients on the ketogenic diet was approximately 78%, but the response rate of patients on the standard diet was only 25%. Progressing disease was 11% in ketogenic diet patients, but it was much higher in standard diet patients (50%). Some of their patients had apparent brief disappearance of tumor tissue.

Schwartz et al. examined the enzyme structures of cancer cells in 17 patients (Schwartz, Noel, Nikolai, & Chang, 2018). They found brain cancer cells lacked enzymes to metabolize ketone bodies. They found evidence of ketone bodies in the brain tumors of the patients who were being treated with a ketogenic diet. The growth of a neuroblastoma was reduced by a ketogenic diet (Weber et al., 2018). They found that an ad lib ketogenic diet 8:1 ratio produced a very strong anti-tumor effect.

For other types of brain cancer such as astrocytoma or medulloblastoma, the effect of a ketogenic diet is less promising (Weber et al., 2018).

Pancreatic Cancer

After patients had surgery for pancreatic-biliary cancer, a ketogenic diet was used instead of the customary high-carbohydrate diet. Patients consumed more calories, had a higher energy intake, and reported more satisfaction with this diet. There were no additional complications (Ok et al., 2018). The authors reported that the ketogenic diet is safe and has potential value as an adjuvant anti-cancer therapy.

Prostate Cancer

The incidence of prostate cancer, the second leading cause of cancer related deaths, varies by nationality. Overall, men in Western countries have a six-times greater rate of prostate cancer than do men in China and Japan. Could the diets of men in China and Japan explain the difference in cancer rates? Animal studies have also shown that mice fed a no-carbohydrate or ketogenic diet had slowed prostate tumor growth and increased survival rates when compared to animals fed a low-fat diet or Western diet.

Most of us couldn't tolerate the very low carbohydrate diet fed to these mice, so the research group looked at several low carbohydrate diets, including the Modified Atkins Diet (MAD). They found that mice consuming diets containing 10 to 20 percent carbohydrates have cancer statistics like those fed a very low carbohydrate diet. The researchers concluded that a less-restrictive low carbohydrate diet might have the same benefits for human patients (Weber et al., 2018).

Ovarian and Endometrial Cancer

For patients with endometrial or ovarian cancer, using a ketogenic diet can improve the patient's quality of life. Patients report improved well-being including reduced insomnia, more energy, decreased appetite, and decreased cravings (Cohen et al., 2018).

Colon Cancer

Colon cancer tumor cells were injected into mice. The mice were fed a ketogenic diet rich in Omega 3, a ketogenic diet with lard, or a standard diet. Both ketogenic diets were associated with slowed tumor growth as compared to the standard diet (Hao et al., 2015).

Stomach, Breast, and Liver Cancer

There is no support for the use of a ketogenic diet as an adjunctive treatment for these cancers (Weber et al., 2018).

Remember, though, the research on the effects of a ketogenic diet on cancer is in its early stages. Many of the studies are animal studies. There is absolutely no evidence that a ketogenic diet cures cancer or that all cancer types will respond to a ketogenic diet in the same way.

Neurological Disorders

The strongest support for the health boosting properties of a ketogenic diet comes from the treatment of neurological illnesses. In fact, the ketogenic diet has been described as neurochemotherapeutic (Veyrat-Durebex et al., 2018). We know more about the efficacy of a ketogenic diet in the treatment of neurological disorders than other diseases due to the application of a ketogenic diet to seizures. The advantages of a ketogenic diet have been studied in animal models of neurological illness as well as human studies. The beneficial effects of a ketogenic diet on a wide range of neurological conditions may stem from the advantage which ketone bodies have in the metabolism of brain cells. Many studies support the notion that cellular energy status is an important factor in multiple neurological disorders. Altered energy production has been linked to epilepsy and Alzheimer's disease.

Intractable Epilepsy

Intractable or refractory epilepsy is defined by inadequate control of seizures despite optimal treatment with conventional medications (Lefevre & Aronson, 2000). Of the 2.5 million patients with epilepsy in the United States, 25% to 30% can be considered to have intractable epilepsy. The efficacy of a ketogenic diet in treatment-resistant epilepsy in children and adults was demonstrated almost a century ago. In the early applications of the low carbohydrate diet, the carbohydrate restrictions were severe. Recently, the Modified Atkins Diet (MAD) was offered to a group of patients with intractable epilepsy. Researchers found that the less restrictive ketogenic diet was easier for patients to follow. Several studies have shown that the MAD is as effective as the classic ketogenic diet for recurrent epileptic seizures (Zhang et al., 2018). The MAD is now the primary option for the treatment of intractable epilepsy in children.

In a recent review of the literature (Liu et al., 2018), the ketogenic diet was effective for adult patients with intractable or treatment resistant epilepsy. Approximately 13% of patients treated with a ketogenic diet became seizure free, and 53% of these patients experienced a smaller number of seizures. Although the energy proportion from the three main nutrient groups— carbohydrates, protein and fat—differed among studies, all the diets were essentially high in fat and low in carbohydrates, forcing the body to use fat as its primary energy source (Guntner et al., 2018).

The mechanism of the effect of ketosis on seizures is not understood. There are several theories.

1. Ketone bodies stabilize the central nervous system.
2. The acidosis which accompanies ketosis modifies the seizure threshold.
3. Changes in fluid and electrolyte balance in the brain modifies the seizure threshold.
4. Change in fat concentration in the blood has an anti-seizure effect.
5. Change in transmitter balance and seizure threshold (Bostock et al., 2017; Veyrat-Durebex et al., 2018).

Elamin and colleagues looked at the impact of a ketogenic diet on the hippocampus (Elamin, Ruskin, Masino, & Sacchetti, 2018). The hippocampus might serve as a seizure gate. A ketogenic diet increases levels of nicotinamine adenine dinucleotide (NAD+). Increased levels of NAD+ protects against the damaging effects of oxidative stress and lengthens the lifespan of nerve cells.

Although the ketogenic diet has been found to be effective in reducing seizures in patients with treatment-refractory epilepsy, less attention has been paid to possible additional cognitive benefits of the diet (van Berkel & Verkuyl, 2018). Using subjective assessments of the patients' experiences, widespread mental or cognitive improvements are reported by patients during treatment with a ketogenic diet. Patients report being more alert, better able to pay attention, and better able to think. When the patients on a ketogenic diet are given standardized tests of mental function, they are more focused while their overall intelligence remains the same. There are indications that these improvements are caused by both seizure reduction and the direct effects of a ketogenic diet on brain function. Wu et al. reported a reduction of 50% or more in seizures, better mental functioning, and improved language skills (Wu et al., 2018).

The effect of following a ketogenic diet on seizure activity is powerful, and mental functioning is improved in most patients (Wu et al., 2018). Patients with intractable epilepsy stay on the ketogenic diet for extended periods of time, and they report mild to no reactions to the diet (Liu et al., 2018).

Glut-1 Deficiency

A Glut-1 deficiency, caused by impaired glucose transport into the brain, is linked to seizures, brain damage, and movement problems. This deficiency can be treated with ketogenic diet therapy (Heussinger et al., 2018). These patients stayed on the ketogenic diet for 10 years, and there were no cardiovascular risks identified in this patient group.

Cluster Migraine Headache

Some people with cluster migraine headaches don't get relief from medication. In one study, following a MAD diet was associated with reduced headache frequency. There were no significant negative effects of following the MAD diet (Di Lorenzo et al., 2018).

Alzheimer's Disease

In a well-controlled study, patients with Alzheimer's disease took an oral ketogenic compound. Daily uses of this compound increased important ketone bodies, and the patients' performances improved on tests of cognition (Bostock et al., 2017).

Ischemic Stroke

Following a ketogenic diet decreases cerebral edema or swelling as well as the size of the brain damage caused by the stroke. It is possible that the beta-hydroxybutyrate ketone body prevents the neuronal cell death caused by glucose deprivation or loss of oxygen. It is also possible that the inflammation associated with stroke is reduced by a ketogenic diet (Guo et al., 2018).

Parkinson's Disease

Preliminary evidence suggests that a low carbohydrate diet can improve the motor and nonmotor symptoms of Parkinson's Disease (Phillips, Murtagh, Gilbertson, Asztely, & Lynch, 2018). Following a ketogenic diet reduces the severity of many symptoms—urinary problems, pain, fatigue, daytime sleepiness, and cognitive impairment. A standard low-fat diet, on the other hand, is associated with only an 11% reduction in symptoms. The investigators speculated that the ketone bodies produced by a high-fat, low-carbohydrate ketogenic diet enhanced the functioning of the mitochondria in the brain and increased the production of new mitochondria. No negative consequences of the ketogenic diet were noted after eight weeks.

Following a ketogenic diet might also benefit patients with motor problems caused by amyotrophic lateral sclerosis, head trauma, and spinal cord injury. The ketogenic diet may change the nerve cells so that they are more efficient (Veyrat-Durebex et al., 2018). Ketogenic diets impact tissues that have high energy requirements. Both the brain and the movement systems require a lot of energy.

Autism Spectrum Disorder (ASD)

We debated about the placement of this discussion. ASD is classified in psychiatric diagnostic manuals, but it is a neurological condition. We decided ASD fits best in the neurological disorder section. The ketogenic diet is emerging as a potential treatment for ASD. Several different diets have been used with ASD patients. These diets are generally having positive results.

Using a ketogenic diet which is low in carbohydrates, moderate in proteins, and uses medium-chain triglyceride oil improves the behavior of ASD patients. The social behavior of these patients is said to be much improved. Fifty percent of the patients were better able to imitate, use their bodies, and were less fearful. The diet is described as a "potentially beneficial option to improve the core features of autism spectrum disorder and warrants further investigation" (Lee et al., 2018).

Psychiatric Disorders

We know much less about the impact of a ketogenic diet on psychiatric conditions because these illnesses have received less attention. Most of the studies are case reports or have limited controls (Bostock et al., 2017). Many of the group studies use animal models of human psychiatric illness. There is a weak link between the anxiety of a mouse and that of you or me. However, due to the strong overlap between neurological and psychiatric illnesses, we can expect more research studies in the future.

Anxiety

Most of the research on the effects of a ketogenic diet on anxiety has been done with animals. In one study, two types of ketone supplements were given to rats. Supplementing the diet increased ketone body levels and produced ketosis. Both conditions reduced the anxiety of rats tested in an elevated maze (Bostock, 2017).

Depression

Adult mice were fed a ketogenic diet during development in utero. These mice were less susceptible to fear and showed increased physical activity (Bostock, 2017).

Bipolar Disorder

Two women with Bipolar Disorder II were followed for several years after starting a ketogenic diet. The women reported that their moods were more stable than when they were taking medication. In another case study, however, the patient didn't benefit from following a ketogenic diet (Bostock et al., 2017).

Schizophrenia

In an animal model of schizophrenia, eating a ketogenic diet reduced the animals' hyperactivity, stereotyped activity, social withdrawal, and working memory deficits. There are a few case studies that report the positive effects of using a ketogenic diet in humans (Bostock et al., 2017).

Attention Deficit Hyperactivity Disorder

There are no clinical studies on Attention Deficit Hyperactivity Disorder. The information we have if based on animal studies. For example, dogs were fed a ketogenic diet. The dogs became less excitable and more trainable over the course of the study (Bostock et al., 2017).

Longevity

In our view, the issue of lifespan tops our list. We all want to live longer and healthier. Eating a ketogenic diet may do both. Most of our understanding of the role that diet has on lifespan comes from animal research. It is well known that reducing the number of calories an organism eats (caloric restriction) makes it live longer on the average. How does eating a ketogenic diet compare to calorie restriction? Do they both improve lifespan? The benefits of caloric restriction and a ketogenic diet are similar. Evidence is now accumulating which suggests that feeding mice a ketogenic diet makes them live longer and function at a higher level (Roberts et al., 2017). If elderly mice are fed a ketogenic diet, their motor skills, memory, and muscle mass are improved. In addition, the mice have better body health markers. In other words, the ketogenic diet slows the aging process for mice. The investigators suggest that ketone bodies protect neurons (Castro et al., 2018).

Conclusions

Each of us has our own level of proof—the level which must be reached before we act. We don't know what your level of proof is, and we're not trying to convince you to follow a low carbohydrate diet to lose weight or to improve your health.

What we can tell you is that a ketogenic diet helped one of us, L. J., lose weight at a rate and with a degree of comfort she didn't expect. We've also decided to continue eating a low carbohydrate diet. We're doing this for two reasons. First, L. J. knows the weight will come back if she starts stuffing down the chocolates and slurping the sodas. The call of the carbohydrate is nearly irresistible to the addict. Second, we believe maintaining a lower body weight may prolong our lives and improve our quality of life. It is our hope and expectation that staying on a keto diet will prevent illness.

Exercise

Decision time. Can you commit to controlling your carbohydrate addiction? This is a life changing decision. Once you accept your addiction, you can never return to your former eating patterns. Like the alcoholic, there is no going back to the old ways.

CHAPTER 23

The future ain't what it used to be. — *Yogi Berra*

Time to Say Goodbye

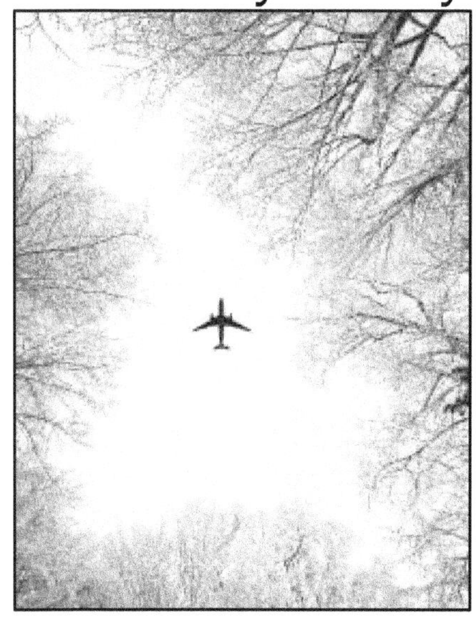

I've been on a low carb diet for 17 months, and I've maintained a stable weight for a year. I've shared everything I know and added Robert's expertise. I know I should write a summary—it's expected. I'm nervous as I try to write this. I want to say just the right thing. I want to say something that will inspire you, the reader, to take a close look at the benefits of living a ketogenic lifestyle. Photo by Oleg Magni from Pexels

We've made several points, each of which clamors for our attention. We thought and thought and decided on two points. First, the central issue for your diet success is finding the right low carbohydrate weight loss program. The mistake I regret most was believing that finding a diet and sticking with it would make me lose weight, i.e., selecting a number of calories consistent with my weight loss goal and expecting to reach that goal. I've learned that diets must be tinkered with, must be adjusted and changed through the diet process. None of us has the objectivity or experience to make these adjustments. What is required is a mentor or a coach, someone who has already accomplished what we hope to accomplish.

We emphasize finding a program with a mentor because following a diet in a book or on the Internet might work for some of us, but not for all of us. You can't talk to the author of a book. A book can't congratulate you when you succeed and encourage when you are low. You can sometimes talk to a counselor if you subscribe to an Internet weight loss program, but you can't know if the counselor is following a script or if the counselor has walked the walk. My counselor was a blessing. She'd walked the walk, and she was cheering for me every step of the way. She had the experience and the objectivity to make suggestions and corrections to my diet. For example, drinking water helps you lose weight. I have a terrible time with this. I think I am descended from camels.

A second important aspect of a weight loss program is medical supervision. This is essential if you have medical issues, as I do. It is particularly important if you have metabolic syndrome. You will probably need to take some supplements as I did. Which supplements?

Why not use your doctor as your weight loss coach? Your doctor may be able to tell you which supplements are safe for you, but doctors are not trained in nutrition or weight loss. Despite the fact that the US Burden of Disease Collaborators identified poor-quality of diet as the leading cause of death in the United States (Devries, Willett, & Bonow, 2019), medical students spend a total of 19 hours studying nutrition. Nutrition education is minimal or missing in most residencies.

Physicians are notorious for preaching health habits they don't follow. Devries et al. asked the question, "Is it appropriate to serve soft drinks and pizza at a resident conference while bemoaning the high prevalence of obesity and encouraging patients to eat healthier?" These authors also note that medical conferences often serve doughnuts and bagels during morning sessions.

Doctors don't necessarily know how to walk the walk. They can, however, help us set goals and monitor our progress. They can also refer us to other professionals such as geneticists for genetic screening, bariatric surgeons, and dietitians.

We wish we could tell you that there's a magic bullet for weight loss. Poof! Fat gone. We want our doctor to pull out a prescription pad and send us to the pharmacy for the magic pill which will cure our ills. I know we want Jenny Craig or Nutrisystem to sell us a few months of food to get those nasty pounds off.

Sadly, diet pills, short-term food interventions, bariatric surgery, or even the best low carbohydrate weight loss program won't address the psychological and addiction issues which we've been discussing in this book. These psychological issues which are part of your personal history as well as carbohydrate addiction are the root causes of your weight problems. Both are inescapable. Both must be addressed to avoid Yo-Yo weight loss and weight regain.

I still struggle with cravings each week, but I am no longer depressed and angry. I am determined. I weigh-in at the center each week, and I weigh myself every three days. I know I must confront my weight to avoid slipping into old patterns and to avoid convincing myself that a few bites of this or that won't hurt. I know I want to trick myself into thinking I'm cured. I'm not. I think I'm winning the battle to accept myself as the carbohydrate addict I am. I still miss some of my food indulgences of the past. I suppose I always will. The way my body feels tells me every day that the struggle has been worth it.

We wish you the best. We'd love to hear from you. Your story is important. We are carb addicts. We are legion.

To be continued?

ABOUT THE AUTHORS

Linda J. Gummow, Ph.D. is a forensic neuropsychologist who lives in Jacksonville, FL with her husband and co-author, R. E. Conger, Ph.D. They had a private practice in Salt Lake City, UT for many years. While Linda specialized in forensic and vocational assessment, Robert worked in a treatment center for behavior disordered children. He treated many children and their families. Both authors have research experience and scientific publications.

Linda also writes mysteries featuring a transgender detective which is set in New Orleans. Her first book, *Unbalanced*, was released in January 2019. The book is available through Amazon.

http://www.amazon.com/dp/B07MDSD7XK

* * * *

Robert is working on a book for parents to help them protect their children from carbohydrate addiction. Contact him with your ideas and suggestions.

* * * *

Robert's email address: robconger8115@gmail.com
Linda's email address: gummowl@yahoo.com
Contact us at our website. We want to hear your stories, comments, suggestions, and criticisms.
Website: https://www.carbohydrateconfessions.com

ABOUT METABOLIC RESEARCH CENTER™

MRC, based in Florida, has been in the business of helping folks like us lose weight for more than 35 years. They offer weight loss services and products in a several states, but your state, city, or town may not have a center. You can enroll in the program online, but if you want to talk to a real-life human, my counselor, Barb Kershner, has given me permission to give her contact information. You may call Barb at (904) 567-9805. Ask for her or leave a message for her. Tell her that you got her name from me. You can get counseling by telephone and products by mail.

REFERENCES

Aaron, D. J., & Hughes, T. L. (2007). Association of childhood sexual abuse with obesity in a community sample of lesbians. *Obesity (Silver Spring), 15*(4), 1023-1028. doi:10.1038/oby.2007.634

Adam, T. C., & Epel, E. S. (2017). Stress, eating and the reward system. *Physiology and Behavior, 91*(4), 449-458.

Adam, T. C., Hasson, R. E., Ventura, E. E., Toledo-Corral, C., Le, K. A., Mahurkar, S.,. Goran, M. I. (2010). Cortisol is negatively associated with insulin sensitivity in overweight Latino youth. *J Clin Endocrinol Metab, 95*(10), 4729-4735. doi:10.1210/jc.2010-0322

Ahmed, S. H., Guillem, K., & Vandaele, Y. (2013). Sugar addiction: pushing the drug-sugar analogy to the limit. *Curr Opin Clin Nutr Metab Care, 16*(4), 434-439. doi:10.1097/MCO.0b013e328361c8b8

Atkins, R. C. (1972). *Dr. Atkins Diet Revoluation*: Bantam Press.

Azad, M. B., Abou-Setta, A. M., Chauhan, B. F., Rabbani, R., Lys, J., Copstein, L., Zarychanski, R. (2017). Nonnutritive sweeteners and cardiometabolic health: a systematic review and meta-analysis of randomized controlled trials and prospective cohort studies. *CMAJ, 189*(28), E929-E939. doi:10.1503/cmaj.161390

Bacon, L. (2008). *Health at every size: The surprising truth about your weight*. Dallas, TX: BenBella.

Bacon, L., Keim, N. L., Van Loan, M. D., Derricote, M., Gale, B., Kazaks, A., & Stern, J. S. (2002). Evaluating a 'non-diet' wellness intervention for improvement of metabolic fitness, psychological well-being and eating and activity behaviors. *Int J Obes Relat Metab Disord, 26*(6), 854-865. doi:10.1038/sj.ijo.0802012

Barnett, R. (2005). Obesity. *Lancet, 366*(9490), 984. doi:10.1016/S0140-6736(05)67376-X

Beavers, K. M., Beavers, D. P., Nesbit, B. A., Ambrosius, W. T., Marsh, A. P., Nicklas, B. J., & Rejeski, W. J. (2014). Effect of an 18-month physical activity and weight loss intervention on body composition in overweight and obese older adults. *Obesity (Silver Spring), 22*(2), 325-331. doi:10.1002/oby.20607

Berridge, K., & E. Robinson, T. (2016). *Liking, wanting, and the incentive-sensitization theory of addiction* (Vol. 71).

Berridge, K. C., & Kringelbach, M. L. (2008). Affective neuroscience of pleasure: reward in humans and animals. *Psychopharmacology, 199*(Three), 457 – 480.

Berridge, K. C., & Robinson, T. E. (2016). Liking, Wanting and the Incentive-Sensitization Theory of Addiction. *The American psychologist, 71*(8), 670-679. doi:10.1037/amp0000059

Blackburn, A. N., Hajnal, A., & Leggio, L. (2017). The gut in the brain: the effects of bariatric surgery on alcohol consumption. *Addict Biol, 22*(6), 1540-1553. doi:10.1111/adb.12436

Bosco, G., Rizzato, A., Quartesan, S., Camporesi, E., Mangar, D., Paganini, M., Paoli, A. (2018). Effects of the Ketogenic diet in overweight divers breathing Enriched Air Nitrox. *Sci Rep, 8*(1), 2655. doi:10.1038/s41598-018-20933-w

Bostock, E. C. S., Kirkby, K. C., & Taylor, B. V. M. (2017). The Current Status of the Ketogenic Diet in Psychiatry. *Frontiers in Psychiatry, 8*(43). doi:10.3389/fpsyt.2017.00043

Brochu, P. M., & Esses, V. M. (2011). What's in a name? The effects of the labels "fat" versus "overweight" on weight bias. *Journal of Applied Social Psychology, 41*(8), 1981-2008.

Buettner, D. (2008). *The Blue Zones*. Washington, D.C.: National Geographical Society.

Carlier, N., Marshe, V. S., Cmorejova, J., Davis, C., & Muller, D. J. (2015). Genetic Similarities between Compulsive Overeating and Addiction Phenotypes: A Case for "Food Addiction"? *Curr Psychiatry Rep, 17*(12), 96. doi:10.1007/s11920-015-0634-5

Castro, A. I., Gomez-Arbelaez, D., Crujeiras, A. B., Granero, R., Aguera, Z., Jimenez-Murcia, S., Casanueva, F. F. (2018). Effect of A Very Low-Calorie Ketogenic Diet on Food and Alcohol Cravings, Physical and Sexual Activity, Sleep Disturbances, and Quality of Life in Obese Patients. *Nutrients, 10*(10). doi:10.3390/nu10101348

Cecil, J. E., Tavendale, R., Watt, P., Hetherington, M. M., & Palmer, C. N. (2008). An obesity-associated FTO gene variant and increased energy intake in children. *N Engl J Med, 359*(24), 2558-2566. doi:10.1056/NEJMoa0803839

Chang, S. H., Freeman, N. L. B., Lee, J. A., Stoll, C. R. T., Calhoun, A. J., Eagon, J. C., & Colditz, G. A. (2018). Early major complications after bariatric surgery in the USA, 2003-2014: a systematic review and meta-analysis. *Obes Rev, 19*(4), 529-537. doi:10.1111/obr.12647

Chao, A. M., Grilo, C. M., & Sinha, R. (2016). Food cravings, binge eating, and eating disorder psychopathology: Exploring the moderating roles of gender and race. *Eat Behav, 21*, 41-47. doi:10.1016/j.eatbeh.2015.12.007

Chao, A. M., White, M. A., Grilo, C. M., & Sinha, R. (2017). Examining the effects of cigarette smoking on food cravings and intake, depressive symptoms, and stress. *Eat Behav, 24*, 61-65. doi:10.1016/j.eatbeh.2016.12.009

Choquet, H., & Meyre, D. (2011). Genetics of Obesity: What have we Learned? *Current Genomics, 12*, 169 – 179.

Cohen, C. W., Fontaine, K. R., Arend, R. C., Soleymani, T., & Gower, B. A. (2018). Favorable Effects of a Ketogenic Diet on Physical Function, Perceived Energy, and Food Cravings in Women with Ovarian or Endometrial Cancer: A Randomized, Controlled Trial. *Nutrients, 10*(9). doi:10.3390/nu10091187

Conradt, M., Dierk, J. M., Schlumberger, P., Rauh, E., Hebebrand, J., & Rief, W. (2007). Development of the Weight- and Body-Related Shame and Guilt scale (WEB-SG) in a nonclinical sample of obese individuals. *J Pers Assess, 88*(3), 317-327. doi:10.1080/00223890701331856

Devries, S., Willett, W., & Bonow, R. O. (2019). Nutrition Education in Medical School, Residency Training, and Practice. *JAMA*. doi:10.1001/jama.2019.1581

Di Lorenzo, C., Coppola, G., Di Lenola, D., Evangelista, M., Sirianni, G., Rossi, P., Pierelli, F. (2018). Efficacy of Modified Atkins Ketogenic Diet in Chronic Cluster Headache: An Open-Label, Single-Arm, Clinical Trial. *Front Neurol, 9*, 64. doi:10.3389/fneur.2018.00064

Dickerson, S. S., Gruenewald, T. L., & Kemeny, M. E. (2004). When the social self is threatened. Shame, physiology, and health. *Journal of Personality, 72*(6), 1191-1216.

Druce, M. R., Small, C. J., & Bloom, S. R. (2004). Minireview: Gut peptides regulating satiety. *Endocrinology, 145*(6), 2660-2665. doi:10.1210/en.2004-0089

DuBreuil, L., Sogg, S. (2017). Alcohol-use disorders after bariatric surgery: The case for targeted group therapy. *Current Psychiatry, 16*(1), 39-49.

El Ghoch, M., Calugi, S., & Dalle Grave, R. (2018). Weight cycling in adults with severe obesity: A longitudinal study. *Nutr Diet, 75*(3), 256-262. doi:10.1111/1747-0080.12387

Elamin, M., Ruskin, D. N., Masino, S. A., & Sacchetti, P. (2018). Ketogenic Diet Modulates NAD(+)-Dependent Enzymes and Reduces DNA Damage in Hippocampus. *Front Cell Neurosci, 12*, 263. doi:10.3389/fncel.2018.00263

Elfhag, K., & Morey, L. C. (2008). Personality traits and eating behavior in the obese. Poor self-control in emotional and external eating but assets in restrained eating. *Eat Behav, 9,* 287-293.

Epel, E. S., Lapidus, R., McEwen, B., & Brownell, K. (2001). Stresss may add bite to appetite in women. A laboratory study of stress-induced cortisol and eating behavior. *Psychoneuroendocrinology, 26*(1), 37-49.

Epel, E. S., & Tomiyama, A. J. (2012). Stress and reward neural networks, eating, and obesity. In K. Brownell & M. S. Gold (Eds.), *Handbook of food and addiction.* Oxford: Oxford University Press.

Ertmans, F., Baeyens, F., & Bergh, V. d. (2002). Food likes and their relative importance in human eating behavior: review and preliminary suggestions for health promotion. *Health and Education Research, 16,* 443-456.

Fan, S. (2013). The Fat Fueled Brain: Unnatural or Advantageous. *Scientific American.*

Farooqi, I. S., Drop, S., Clements, A., Keogh, J. M., Biernacka, J., Lowenbein, S., O'Rahilly, S. (2006). Heterozygosity for a POMC-null mutation and increased obesity risk in humans. *Diabetes, 55*(9), 2549-2553. doi:10.2337/db06-0214

Friedman, J. M. (2004). Modern science versus the stigma of obesity. *Nat Med, 10*(6), 563-569. doi:10.1038/nm0604-563

Gahche, J. B., R., Burt, V., Hughes, J., McDowell, M., Sempos, C. (2011). *Dietary Supplement Use Among U. S. Adults Has Increased Since NHANES III (1988-1994).* Hyattsville, MD: National Center for Health Statistic.

Gardner, C. D., Kiazand, A., Alhassan, S., Kim, S., Stafford, R. S., Balise, R. R., . . . King, A. C. (2007). Comparison of the Atkins, Zone, Ornish, and LEARN diets for change in weight and related risk factors among overweight premenopausal women: the A TO Z Weight Loss Study: a randomized trial. *JAMA, 297*(9), 969-977. doi:10.1001/jama.297.9.969

Gearhardt, A. N., Corbin, W. R., & Brownell, K. D. (2009). Preliminary validation of the Yale Food Addiction Scale. *Appetite, 52*(2), 430-436. doi:10.1016/j.appet.2008.12.003

Gerlach, G., Herpertz, S., & Loeber, S. (2015). Personality traits and obesity: a systematic review. *Obes Rev, 16*(1), 32-63. doi:10.1111/obr.12235

Gordon, E. L., Ariel-Donges, A. H., Bauman, V., & Merlo, L. J. (2018). What Is the Evidence for "Food Addiction?" A Systematic Review. *Nutrients, 10*(4), 477. doi:10.3390/nu10040477

Green, E., & Murphy, C. (2012). Altered processing of sweet taste in the brain of diet soda drinkers. *Physiology & behavior, 107*(4), 560-567. doi:10.1016/j.physbeh.2012.05.006

Greenberg, B. S., Eastin, M., Hofschire, L., Lachlan, K., & Brownell, K. D. (2003). Portrayals of overweight and obese individuals on commercial television. *Am J Public Health, 93*(8), 1342-1348.

Greeno, C. G., & Wing, R. R. (1994). Stress induced eating. *Psychological Bulletin, 115*(3), 444-464.

Greenway, F. L., Fujioka, K., Plodkowski, R. A., Mudaliar, S., Guttadauria, M., Erickson, J., Group, C.-I. S. (2010). Effect of naltrexone plus bupropion on weight loss in overweight and obese adults (COR-I): a multicentre, randomised, double-blind, placebo-controlled, phase 3 trial. *Lancet, 376*(9741), 595-605. doi:10.1016/S0140-6736(10)60888-4

Gregorio, V. D., Lucchese, R., Vera, I., Silva, G. C., Silva, A., & Moraes, R. C. (2016). The Alcohol Consumption Is Amended after Bariatric Surgery? An Integrative Review. *Arq Bras Cir Dig, 29Suppl* 1(Suppl 1), 111-115. doi:10.1590/0102-6720201600S10027

Gudzune, K. A., Doshi, R. S., Mehta, A. K., Chaudhry, Z. W., Jacobs, D. K., Vakil, R. M., . . . Clark, J. M. (2015). Efficacy of commercial weight loss programs: an updated systematic review. *Annals of Internal Medicine, 162*(7), 501-512. doi:10.7326/M14-2238

Guntner, A. T., Kompalla, J. F., Landis, H., Theodore, S. J., Geidl, B., Sievi, N. A., Gerber, P. A. (2018). Guiding Ketogenic Diet with Breath Acetone Sensors. *Sensors (Basel), 18*(11). doi:10.3390/s18113655

Guo, M., Wang, X., Zhao, Y., Yang, Q., Ding, H., Dong, Q.,. Cui, M. (2018). Ketogenic Diet Improves Brain Ischemic Tolerance and Inhibits NLRP3 Inflammasome Activation by Preventing Drp1-Mediated Mitochondrial Fission and Endoplasmic Reticulum Stress. *Front Mol Neurosci, 11,* 86. doi:10.3389/fnmol.2018.00086

Hao, G. W., Chen, Y. S., He, D. M., Wang, H. Y., Wu, G. H., & Zhang, B. (2015). Growth of human colon cancer cells in nude mice is delayed by ketogenic diet with or without omega-3 fatty acids and medium-chain triglycerides. *Asian Pac J Cancer Prev, 16*(5), 2061-2068.

Haraguchi, A., Fukuzawa, M., Iwami, S., Nishimura, Y., Motohashi, H., Tahara, Y., & Shibata, S. (2018). Night eating model shows time-specific depression-like behavior in the forced swimming test. *Sci Rep, 8*(1), 1081. doi:10.1038/s41598-018-19433-8

Harrison, K. (2000). Television viewing, fat stereotyping, body shape standards, and eating disordered symptomatology in grade school children. *Communication Research, 27,* 617-640.

Hebebrand, J., Albayrak, O., Adan, R., Antel, J., Dieguez, C., de Jong, J., Dickson, S. L. (2014). "Eating addiction", rather than "food addiction", better captures addictive-like eating behavior. *Neurosci Biobehav Rev, 47,* 295-306. doi:10.1016/j.neubiorev.2014.08.016

Hemmingsson, E. (2018). Early Childhood Obesity Risk Factors: Socioeconomic Adversity, Family Dysfunction, Offspring Distress, and Junk Food Self-Medication. *Curr Obes Rep, 7*(2), 204-209. doi:10.1007/s13679-018-0310-2

Hemmingsson, E., Johansson, K., & Reynisdottir, S. (2014). Effects of childhood abuse on adult obesity: a systematic review and meta-analysis. *Obes Rev, 15*(11), 882-893. doi:10.1111/obr.12216

Henderson, B. (2018). The Murdock Study. *Tribune News Service.*

Heussinger, N., Della Marina, A., Beyerlein, A., Leiendecker, B., Hermann-Alves, S., Dalla Pozza, R., & Klepper, J. (2018). 10 patients, 10 years - Long term follow-up of cardiovascular risk factors in Glut1 deficiency treated with ketogenic diet therapies: A prospective, multicenter case series. *Clin Nutr, 37*(6 Pt A), 2246-2251. doi:10.1016/j.clnu.2017.11.001

Himes, S. M., & Thompson, J. K. (2007). Fat stigmatization in television shows and movies: a content analysis. *Obesity (Silver Spring), 15*(3), 712-718. doi:10.1038/oby.2007.635

Hinney, A., Vogel, C. I., & Hebebrand, J. (2010). From monogenic to polygenic obesity: recent advances. *Eur Child Adolesc Psychiatry, 19*(3), 297-310. doi:10.1007/s00787-010-0096-6

Hoogeveen, H. R., Jolij, J., Ter Horst, G. J., & Lorist, M. M. (2016). Brain Potentials Highlight Stronger Implicit Food Memory for Taste than Health and Context Associations. *PLOs One, 11*(5), e0154128. doi:10.1371/journal.pone.0154128

Horstmann, A., Dietrich, A., Mathar, D., Possel, M., Villringer, A., & Neumann, J. (2015). Slave to habit? Obesity is associated with decreased behavioural sensitivity to reward devaluation. *Appetite, 87,* 175-183. doi:10.1016/j.appet.2014.12.212

Hsu, A., Yang, J., Yilmaz, Y., Haque, S., Cengiz, C., & Blanford, A. (2014). Persuasive technology for overcoming food cravings and improving snack choices. Retrieved from http://dl.//.acm.org/citation.cfm?id+2557099*

Hulbert-Williams, L., Hulbert-Williams, N. J., Nicholls, W., Williamson, S., Poonia, J., & Hochard, K. D. (2017). Ultra-brief non-expert-delivered defusion and acceptance exercises for food cravings: A partial replication study. *J Health Psychol*, 1359105317695424. doi:10.1177/1359105317695424

Hunger, J. M., & Tomiyama, A. J. (2014). Weight labeling and obesity: a longitudinal study of girls aged 10 to 19 years. *JAMA Pediatr, 168*(6), 579-580. doi:10.1001/jamapediatrics.2014.122

Hyman, R. J. (2001). *Asparame Disease: An Ignored Epidemic*. Palm Beach, FL: Sunshine Sentinel Press, West.

Hymowitz, G., Salwen, J., & Salis, K. L. (2017). A mediational model of obesity related disordered eating: The roles of childhood emotional abuse and self-perception. *Eat Behav, 26*, 27-32. doi:10.1016/j.eatbeh.2016.12.010

Iacovides, S., & Meiring, R. M. (2018). The effect of a ketogenic diet versus a high-carbohydrate, low-fat diet on sleep, cognition, thyroid function, and cardiovascular health independent of weight loss: study protocol for a randomized controlled trial. *Trials, 19*(1), 62. doi:10.1186/s13063-018-2462-5

Imperatori, C., Fabbricatore, M., Innamorati, M., Farina, B., Quintiliani, M. I., Lamis, D. A., Della Marca, G. (2015). Modification of EEG functional connectivity and EEG power spectra in overweight and obese patients with food addiction: An eLORETA study. *Brain Imaging Behav, 9*(4), 703-716. doi:10.1007/s11682-014-9324-x

Incollingo Rodriguez, A. C., Heldreth, C. M., & Tomiyama, A. J. (2016). Putting on weight stigma: A randomized study of the effects of wearing a fat suit on eating, well-being, and cortisol. *Obesity (Silver Spring), 24*(9), 1892-1898. doi:10.1002/oby.21575

James, B. L., Roe, L. S., Loken, E., & Rolls, B. J. (2018). Early predictors of weight loss in a 1-year behavioural weight loss programme. *Obes Sci Pract, 4*(1), 20-28. doi:10.1002/osp4.149

Joyner, M. A., Kim, S., & Gearhardt, A. N. (2017). Investigating an incentive-sensitzation model of eating behavior: Impat of simulated fast-food laboratpru. *Clinical Psychological Science, 5*(6), 1014-1026.

Kaiser, C. R., Vick, S. B., & Major, B. (2006). Prejudice expectations moderate preconscious attention to cues that are threatening to social identity. *Psychologial Science, 17*(4), 332-338.

Kapoor, E., Collazo-Clavell, M. L., & Faubion, S. S. (2017). Weight Gain in Women at Midlife: A Concise Review of the Pathophysiology and Strategies for Management. *Mayo Clin Proc, 92*(10), 1552-1558. doi:10.1016/j.mayocp.2017.08.004

Karfopoulou, E., Anastasiou, C. A., Avgeraki, E., Kosmidis, M. H., & Yannakoulia, M. (2016). The role of social support in weight loss maintenance: results from the MedWeight study. *J Behav Med, 39*(3), 511-518. doi:10.1007/s10865-016-9717-y

Kephart, W. C., Pledge, C. D., Roberson, P. A., Mumford, P. W., Romero, M. A., Mobley, C. B., . . . Roberts, M. D. (2018). The Three-Month Effects of a Ketogenic Diet on Body Composition, Blood Parameters, and Performance Metrics in CrossFit Trainees: A Pilot Study. *Sports (Basel), 6*(1). doi:10.3390/sports6010001

Konturek, P. C., Konturek, J. W., Czesnikiewicz-Guzik, M., Brzozowski, T., Sito, E., & Konturek, S. J. (2005). Neuro-hormonal control of food intake: basic mechanisms and clinical implications. *J Physiol Pharmacol, 56 Suppl 6*, 5-25.

Kossoff, E. H., & Dorward, J. L. (2008). The Modified Atkins Diet. *Epilepsia Open, 49*, 37-41.

Kozak, A. T., Davis, J., Brown, R., & Grabowski, M. (2017). Are overeating and food addiction related to distress tolerance? An examination of residents with obesity from a U.S. metropolitan area. *Obes Res Clin Pract, 11*(3), 287-298. doi:10.1016/j.orcp.2016.09.010

Kumar, B. N., Meyer, H.E., Wandel, M., Dalen, I., Holmboe-Ottesen, G. (2006). Ethnic Differences in obesity among immigrants from developing countries, in Oslo, Norway. *Int. J. Obes., 30*, 684-690.

Lee, R. W. Y., Corley, M. J., Pang, A., Arakaki, G., Abbott, L., Nishimoto, M., Wong, M. (2018). A modified ketogenic gluten-free diet with MCT improves behavior in children with autism spectrum disorder. *Physiol Behav, 188*, 205-211. doi:10.1016/j.physbeh.2018.02.006

Lefevre, F., & Aronson, N. (2000). Ketogenic diet for the treatment of refractory epilepsy in children: A systematic review of efficacy. *Pediatrics, 105*(4), E46.

Lennerz, B., & Lennerz, J. K. (2018). Food Addiction, High-Glycemic-Index Carbohydrates, and Obesity. *Clin Chem, 64*(1), 64-71. doi:10.1373/clinchem.2017.273532

Lenoir, M., & Fuschia, S. (2007). Intense Sweetness Surpasses Cocaine Reward. *American Journal of Clinical Nutrition, PLOS One.* doi:10:1371/journal.pone.0000698

Li, R., Serdula, M. K., Williamson, D. F., Bowman, B. A., Graham, D. J., & Green, L. (1999). Dose-effect of fenfluramine use on the severity of valvular heart disease among fen-phen patients with valvulopathy. *Int J Obes Relat Metab Disord, 23*(9), 926-928.

Lin, S., Naseri, T., Linhart, C., Morrell, S., Taylor, R., McGarvey, S. T., Zimmet, P. (2017). Trends in diabetes and obesity in Samoa over 35 years, 1978–2013. *Diabetic Medicine, 34*(5), 654-661. doi:10.1111/dme.13197

Liu, H., Yang, Y., Wang, Y., Tang, H., Zhang, F., Zhang, Y., & Zhao, Y. (2018). Ketogenic diet for treatment of intractable epilepsy in adults: A meta-analysis of observational studies. *Epilepsia Open, 3*(1), 9-17. doi:10.1002/epi4.12098

Longo, D. L. (2018). *Longevity Diet.* New York, NY: Penguin.

Ludwig, D. S. (2016). *Alwlays Hungry* (Vol. Always Hungry? Hachette Book Group, NY/NY.

Mackie, G. M., Samocha-Bonet, D., & Tam, C. S. (2017). Does weight cycling promote obesity and metabolic risk factors? *Obes Res Clin Pract, 11*(2), 131-139. doi:10.1016/j.orcp.2016.10.284

MacMillan, S. (2001). *Fit over forty: The winning way to lifetime fitness.* Vancouver, WA: Rain Coast Books.

Madigan, C. D., Pavey, T., Daley, A. J., Jolly, K., & Brown, W. J. (2018). Is weight cycling associated with adverse health outcomes? A cohort study. *Prev Med, 108*, 47-52. doi:10.1016/j.ypmed.2017.12.010

Major, B., Eliezer, D., & Rieck, H. (2012). The psychological weight of weight stigma. *Social Psychology and Personality Science, 3*, 651-658.

Markus, C. R., Rogers, P. J., Brouns, F., & Schepers, R. (2017). Eating dependence and weight gain; no human evidence for a 'sugar-addiction' model of overweight. *Appetite, 114*, 64-72. doi:10.1016/j.appet.2017.03.024

Martin-McGill, K. J., Marson, A. G., Tudur Smith, C., & Jenkinson, M. D. (2018). The Modified Ketogenic Diet in Adults with Glioblastoma: An Evaluation of Feasibility and Deliverability within the National Health Service. *Nutr Cancer, 70*(4), 643-649. doi:10.1080/01635581.2018.1460677

Masko, E. M., Thomas, J. A., 2nd, Antonelli, J. A., Lloyd, J. C., Phillips, T. E., Poulton, S. H., . . . Freedland, S. J. (2010). Low-carbohydrate diets and prostate cancer: how low is "low enough"? *Cancer prevention research (Philadelphia, Pa.)*, 3(9), 1124-1131. doi:10.1158/1940-6207.CAPR-10-0071

McClelland, A., Kemps, E., & Tiggemann, M. (2006). Reduction of vividness and associated craving in personalized food imagery. *J Clin Psychol*, 62(3), 355-365. doi:10.1002/jclp.20216

Meule, A. (2018). Food cravings in food addiction: exploring a potential cut-off value of the Food Cravings Questionnaire-Trait-reduced. *Eat Weight Disord*, 23(1), 39-43. doi:10.1007/s40519-017-0452-3

Meule, A., de Zwaan, M., & Muller, A. (2017). Attentional and motor impulsivity interactively predict 'food addiction' in obese individuals. *Compr Psychiatry*, 72, 83-87. doi:10.1016/j.comppsych.2016.10.001

Meule, A., Richard, A., & Platte, P. (2017). Food cravings prospectively predict decreases in perceived self-regulatory success in dieting. *Eat Behav*, 24, 34-38. doi:10.1016/j.eatbeh.2016.11.007

Minger, D. (2007). *Death by the Food Pyramid*. Malibu California: Primal Blueprint Printing.

Mossle, T., Kliem, S., Lohmann, A., Bergmann, M. C., & Baier, D. (2017). Differential Influences of Parenting Dimensions and Parental Physical Abuse during Childhood on Overweight and Obesity in Adolescents. *Children (Basel)*, 4(3). doi:10.3390/children4030017

Munro, I. A., Bore, M. R., Munro, D., & Garg, M. L. (2011). Using personality as a predictor of diet induced weight loss and weight management. *Int J Behav Nutr Phys Act*, 8, 129. doi:10.1186/1479-5868-8-129

Myers, K. (2015). Why Do We Eat What We Eat? In N. Avena (Ed.), *Hedonic Eating: How the Pleasureable Aspects of Food Can Affect Appetite* (pp. 9-38). New York: Oxford University Press.

Nance, K., Eagon, J. C., Klein, S., & Pepino, M. Y. (2017). Effects of Sleeve Gastrectomy vs. Roux-en-Y Gastric Bypass on Eating Behavior and Sweet Taste Perception in Subjects with Obesity. *Nutrients*, 10(1). doi:10.3390/nu10010018

Nestle, M. (2002). *Food Politics: How the Food Industry Influences Nutrition and Health*. Berkeley: University of California.

Nguyen, H. Q., Maciejewski, M. L., Gao, S., Lin, E., Williams, B., & Logerfo, J. P. (2008). Health care use and costs associated with use of a health club membership benefit in older adults with diabetes. *Diabetes Care*, 31, 1562-1567.

Noll, J. G., Zeller, M. H., Trickett, P. K., & Putnam, F. W. (2007). Obesity risk for female victims of childhood sexual abuse: a prospective study. *Pediatrics*, 120(1), e61-67. doi:10.1542/peds.2006-3058

O'Rahilly, S., & Farooqi, I. S. (2008). Human obesity: a heritable neurobehavioral disorder that is highly sensitive to environmental conditions. *Diabetes*, 57(11), 2905-2910. doi:10.2337/db08-0210

Ochner, C. N., Laferrère, B., Afifi, L., Atalayer, D., Pantazatos, S. P., Geliebter, A., Hirsch, J. (2012). Neural Responsivity to Food Cues in Fasted and Fed States Pre and Post Gastric Bypass Surgery. *Neuroscience research*, 74(2), 138-143. doi:10.1016/j.neures.2012.08.002

Ok, J. H., Lee, H., Chung, H. Y., Lee, S. H., Choi, E. J., Kang, C. M., & Lee, S. M. (2018). The Potential Use of a Ketogenic Diet in Pancreatobiliary Cancer Patients After Pancreatectomy. *Anticancer Res*, 38(11), 6519-6527. doi:10.21873/anticanres.13017

Oldham, M., Tomiyama, A. J., & Robinson, E. (2018). The psychosocial experience of feeling overweight promotes increased snack food consumption in women but not men. *Appetite*, 128, 283-293. doi:10.1016/j.appet.2018.05.002

Olds, J., & Milner, P. (1954). Positive reinforcement produced by electrical stimulation of septal area and other regions of rat brain. *J Comp Physiol Psychol, 47*(6), 419-427.

Olejniczak, D., Bugajec, D., Staniszewska, A., Panczyk, M., Kielan, A., Czerw, A., Brytek-Matera, A. (2018). Risk assessment of night-eating syndrome occurrence in women in Poland, considering the obesity factor in particular. *Neuropsychiatr Dis Treat, 14*, 1521-1526. doi:10.2147/NDT.S159562

Palm, I. F., Schram, R., Swarts, H. J. M., van Schothorst, E. M., & Keijer, J. (2017). Body Weight Cycling with Identical Diet Composition Does Not Affect Energy Balance and Has No Adverse Effect on Metabolic Health Parameters. *Nutrients, 9*(10). doi:10.3390/nu9101149

Paoli, A. (2014). Ketogenic Diet for Obesity: Friend or Foe? *International Journal of Environmental Research and Public Health, 11*(2), 2092 – 2107.

Paoli, A., Bianco, A., Grimaldi, K. A., Lodi, A., & Bosco, G. (2013). Long term successful weight loss with a combination biphasic ketogenic Mediterranean diet and Mediterranean diet maintenance protocol. *Nutrients, 5*(12), 5205-5217. doi:10.3390/nu5125205

Pecoraro, N., Reyes, F., Gomez, F., Bhargava, A., & Dallman, M. F. (2004). Chronic stress promotes palatable feeding, which reduces signs of stress. Feedforward and feedback effects of chronic stress. *Endocrinology, 145*(8), 3754-3762.

Peters, J. C., Marker, R., Pan, Z., Breen, J. A., & Hill, J. O. (2018). The Influence of Adding Spices to Reduced Sugar Foods on Overall Liking. *Journal of Food Science, 83*(3), 814-821. doi:10.1111/1750-3841.14069

Phillips, M. C. L., Murtagh, D. K. J., Gilbertson, L. J., Asztely, F. J. S., & Lynch, C. D. P. (2018). Low-fat versus ketogenic diet in Parkinson's disease: A pilot randomized controlled trial. *Mov Disord, 33*(8), 1306-1314. doi:10.1002/mds.27390

Pinhas-Hamiel, O., Modan-Moses, D., Herman-Raz, M., & Reichman, B. (2009). Obesity in girls and penetrative sexual abuse in childhood. *Acta Paediatr, 98*(1), 144-147. doi:10.1111/j.1651-2227.2008.01044.x

Polk, S. E., Schulte, E. M., Furman, C. R., & Gearhardt, A. N. (2017). Wanting and liking: Separable components in problematic eating behavior? *Appetite, 115*, 45-53. doi:10.1016/j.appet.2016.11.015

Provencher, V., Begin, C., Tremblay, A., Mongeau, L., Corneau, L., Dodin, S., Lemieux, S. (2009). Health-At-Every-Size and eating behaviors: 1-year follow-up results of a size acceptance intervention. *J Am Diet Assoc, 109*(11), 1854-1861. doi:10.1016/j.jada.2009.08.017

Puhl, R. M., Himmelstein, M. S., & Quinn, D. M. (2018). Internalizing Weight Stigma: Prevalence and Sociodemographic Considerations in US Adults. *Obesity (Silver Spring), 26*(1), 167-175. doi:10.1002/oby.22029

Qi, L., Kraft, P., Hunter, D. J., & Hu, F. B. (2008). The common obesity variant near MC4R gene is associated with higher intakes of total energy and dietary fat, weight change and diabetes risk in women. *Hum Mol Genet, 17*(22), 3502-3508. doi:10.1093/hmg/ddn242

Rasmussen, N. (2008). America's first amphetamine epidemic 1929-1971: a quantitative and qualitative retrospective with implications for the present. *American journal of public health, 98*(6), 974-985. doi:10.2105/AJPH.2007.110593

Reinehr, T., Kleber, M., & Toschke, A. M. (2009). Lifestyle intervention in obese children is associated with a decrease of the metabolic syndrome prevalence. *Atherosclerosis, 207*(1), 174-180. doi:10.1016/j.atherosclerosis.2009.03.041

Reinehr, T., Schmidt, C., Toschke, A. M., & Andler, W. (2009). Lifestyle intervention in obese children with non-alcoholic fatty liver disease: 2-year follow-up study. *Arch Dis Child, 94*(6), 437-442. doi:10.1136/adc.2008.143594

Rhee, E. J. (2017). Weight Cycling and its metabolic impact. *Journal of Obesity & Metabolic Syndrome, 26*, 237-242.

Richardson, A. S., Dietz, W. H., & Gordon-Larsen, P. (2014). The association between childhood sexual and physical abuse with incident adult severe obesity across 13 years of the National Longitudinal Study of Adolescent Health. *Pediatr Obes, 9*(5), 351-361. doi:10.1111/j.2047-6310.2013.00196.x

Roberts, M. N., Wallace, M. A., Tomilov, A. A., Zhou, Z., Marcotte, G. R., Tran, D., . . . Lopez-Dominguez, J. A. (2017). A Ketogenic Diet Extends Longevity and Healthspan in Adult Mice. *Cell Metab, 26*(3), 539-546 e535. doi:10.1016/j.cmet.2017.08.005

Robin, M. M. (2014). *Our Daily Poison*. New York, NY: The New Press.

Roza, O., Lovász, N., Zupkó, I., Hohmann, J., & Csupor, D. (2013). Sympathomimetic activity of a Hoodia gordonii product: a possible mechanism of cardiovascular side effects. *BioMed research international, 2013*, 171059-171059. doi:10.1155/2013/171059

Rubin, G. (2017). *The Four Tendencies*. New York: Harmony Books.

Rudenga, K. J., & Small, D. M. (2012). Amygdala response to sucrose consumption is inversely related to artificial sweetener use. *Appetite, 58*(2), 504-507. doi:10.1016/j.appet.2011.12.001

Santos, J. G., Da Cruz, W. M. S., Schonthal, A. H., Salazar, M. D., Fontes, C. A. P., Quirico-Santos, T., & Da Fonseca, C. O. (2018). Efficacy of a ketogenic diet with concomitant intranasal perillyl alcohol as a novel strategy for the therapy of recurrent glioblastoma. *Oncol Lett, 15*(1), 1263-1270. doi:10.3892/ol.2017.7362

Sawamoto, R. (2015). Predictors of drop out of female obese patients treated with group cognitive behavioral therapy. *European Journal of Obesity, 9*, 29-38.

Schmidt, J., & Martin, A. (2017). "Smile away your cravings" - Facial feedback modulates cue-induced food cravings. *Appetite, 116*, 536-543. doi:10.1016/j.appet.2017.05.037

Schvey, N. A., Puhl, R. M., & Brownell, K. D. (2014). The stress of stigma: exploring the effect of weight stigma on cortisol reactivity. *Psychosom Med, 76*(2), 156-162. doi:10.1097/PSY.0000000000000031

Schwartz, K. A., Noel, M., Nikolai, M., & Chang, H. T. (2018). Investigating the Ketogenic Diet As Treatment for Primary Aggressive Brain Cancer: Challenges and Lessons Learned. *Front Nutr, 5*, 11. doi:10.3389/fnut.2018.00011

Shai, I., Schwarzfuchs, D., Henkin, Y., Shahar, D. R., Witkow, S., Greenberg, I., . . . Dietary Intervention Randomized Controlled Trial, G. (2008). Weight loss with a low-carbohydrate, Mediterranean, or low-fat diet. *N Engl J Med, 359*(3), 229-241. doi:10.1056/NEJMoa0708681

Shillito, J. A., Lea, J., Tierney, S., Cleator, J., Tai, S., & Wilding, J. P. H. (2018). Why I eat at night: A qualitative exploration of the development, maintenance and consequences of Night Eating Syndrome. *Appetite, 125*, 270-277. doi:10.1016/j.appet.2018.02.005

Simons, J. S., Gaher, R. M., Oliver, M. N., Bush, J. A., & Palmer, M. A. (2005). An experience sampling study of associations between affect and alcohol use and problems among college students. *J Stud Alcohol, 66*(4), 459-469.

Skorka-Brown, J., Andrade, J., Whalley, B., & May, J. (2015). Playing Tetris decreases drug and other cravings in real world settings. *Addict Behav, 51*, 165-170. doi:10.1016/j.addbeh.2015.07.020

Stryjecki, C., Alyass, A., & Meyre, D. (2018). Ethnic and population differences in the genetic predisposition to human obesity. *Obes Rev, 19*(1), 62-80. doi:10.1111/obr.12604

Stunkard, A., & Lu, X. Y. (2010). Rapid changes in night eating: considering mechanisms. *Eat Weight Disord, 15*(1-2), e2-8.

Stunkard, A. J., Foch, T. T., & Hrubec, Z. (1986). A twin study of human obesity. *JAMA, 256*(1), 51-54.

Stunkard, A. J., Harris, J. R., Pedersen, N. L, McClearn, G. E. (1990). The body-mass index of twins who have been reared apart. *N. Engl. J. Med., 322*, 1483-1487.

Suez, J., Korem, T., Zeevi, D., Zilberman-Schapira, G., Thaiss, C. A., Maza, O., Elinav, E. (2014). Artificial sweeteners induce glucose intolerance by altering the gut microbiota. *Nature, 514*(7521), 181-186. doi:10.1038/nature13793

Sutin, A. R., & Terracciano, A. (2013). Perceived weight discrimination and obesity. *PLOs One, 8*(7). doi:10.1371/journal.pone.0070048

Swithers, S. E., Baker, C. R., & Davidson, T. L. (2009). General and persistent effects of high-intensity sweeteners on body weight gain and caloric compensation in rats. *Behav Neurosci, 123*(4), 772-780. doi:10.1037/a0016139

Swithers, S. E., & Davidson, T. L. (2008). A role for sweet taste: calorie predictive relations in energy regulation by rats. *Behav Neurosci, 122*(1), 161-173. doi:10.1037/0735-7044.122.1.161

Taubes, G. (2001). Nutrition. The soft science of dietary fat. *Science, 291*(5513), 2536-2545.

Teicholz, N. (2014). *The Big Fat Surprise*. New York, N. Y.: Simon and Schuster.

Teixeira, J., Going, S. B., Houtkooper, L. B., Cussler, E. C., Martin, C. J., Metcalfe, L. L., Lohman, T. G. (2002). Weight loss readiness in middle-aged women: Psychosocial predictors of success for behavioral weight reduction. *Journal of Behavioral Medicine, 25*(6), 499-523.

Teixeira, P. J., Going, S. B., Houtkooper, L. B., Cussler, E. C., Metcalfe, L. L., Blew, R. M., Lohman, T. G. (2004). Pretreatment predictors of attrition and successful weight management in women. *Int J Obes Relat Metab Disord, 28*(9), 1124-1133. doi:10.1038/sj.ijo.0802727

Teixeira, P. J., Palmeira, A. L., Branco, T. L., Martins, S. S., Minderico, C. S., Barata, J. T., Sardinha, L. B. (2004). Who will lose weight? A reexamination of predictors of weight loss in women. *Int J Behav Nutr Phys Act, 1*(1), 12. doi:10.1186/1479-5868-1-12

Tomiyama, A. J. (2014). Weight stigma is stressful. A review of evidence for the Cyclic Obesity/Weight-Based Stigma model. *Appetite, 82*, 8-15. doi:10.1016/j.appet.2014.06.108

Tomiyama, A. J., & Mann, T. (2013). If shaming reduced obesity, there would be no fat people. *The Hastings Center Report, 43*(3).

Tomlimson, T. (2019). *The Elelphant in the Room: One Fat Man's Quest to Get Smaller in a Growing America*. New York: Simon & Schuster Inc.

Tsai, A. G., Wadden, T. A., Womble, L. G., & Byrne, K. J. (2005). Commercial and self-help programs for weight control. *Psychiatr Clin North Am, 28*(1), 171-192, ix. doi:10.1016/j.psc.2004.10.003

van Berkel, A. A., DM, I. J., & Verkuyl, J. M. (2018). Cognitive benefits of the ketogenic diet in patients with epilepsy: A systematic overview. *Epilepsy Behav, 87*, 69-77. doi:10.1016/j.yebeh.2018.06.004

VanderBroek-Stice, L., Stojek, M. K., Beach, S. R., vanDellen, M. R., & MacKillop, J. (2017). Multidimensional assessment of impulsivity in relation to obesity and food addiction. *Appetite, 112*, 59-68. doi:10.1016/j.appet.2017.01.009

Vargas, S., Romance, R., Petro, J. L., Bonilla, D. A., Galancho, I., Espinar, S., . . . Benitez-Porres, J. (2018). Efficacy of ketogenic diet on body composition during resistance training in trained men: a randomized controlled trial. *J Int Soc Sports Nutr, 15*(1), 31. doi:10.1186/s12970-018-0236-9

Vermaak, I., Hamman, J. H., & Viljoen, A. M. (2011). Hoodia gordonii: an up-to-date review of a commercially important anti-obesity plant. *Planta Med, 77*(11), 1149-1160. doi:10.1055/s-0030-1250643

Veyrat-Durebex, C., Reynier, P., Procaccio, V., Hergesheimer, R., Corcia, P., Andres, C. R., & Blasco, H. (2018). How Can a Ketogenic Diet Improve Motor Function? *Front Mol Neurosci, 11*, 15. doi:10.3389/fnmol.2018.00015

Villareal, D. T., Aguirre, L., Gurney, A. B., Waters, D. L., Sinacore, D. R., Colombo, E., . . . Qualls, C. (2017). Aerobic or Resistance Exercise, or Both, in Dieting Obese Older Adults. *The New England journal of medicine, 376*(20), 1943-1955. doi:10.1056/NEJMoa1616338

Villareal, D. T., Chode, S., Parimi, N., Sinacore, D. R., Hilton, T., Armamento-Villareal, R., . . . Shah, K. (2011). Weight loss, exercise, or both and physical function in obese older adults. *N Engl J Med, 364*(13), 1218-1229. doi:10.1056/NEJMoa1008234

Volkow, N. D., Wang, G. J., Fowler, J. S., Tomasi, D., & Baler, R. (2012). Food and drug reward: overlapping circuits in human obesity and addiction. *Curr Top Behav Neurosci, 11*, 1-24. doi:10.1007/7854_2011_169

Wang, L., Southerland, J., Wang, K., Bailey, B. A., Alamian, A., Stevens, M. A., & Wang, Y. (2017). Ethnic Differences in Risk Factors for Obesity among Adults in California, the United States. *J Obes, 2017*, 2427483. doi:10.1155/2017/2427483

Wansink, B., Cheney, M. M., & Chan, N. (2003). Exploring comfort food preferences across age and gender. *Physiol Behav, 79*(4-5), 739-747.

Waters, D. L. (2013). Weight loss in obese adults 65 years and older: a review of the controversy. *Exp. Gerontol., 48*, 1054-1061.

Weber, D. D., Aminazdeh-Gohari, S., & Kofler, B. (2018). Ketogenic diet in cancer therapy. *Aging (Albany NY), 10*(2), 164-165. doi:10.18632/aging.101382

Westman, E., Phinney, S., & Volek, J. (2010). *New Atkins for a New You*. New York, New York: Simon and Schuster.

White, M. A., McKee, S. A., & O'Malley S, S. (2007). Smoke and mirrors: magnified beliefs that cigarette smoking suppresses weight. *Addict Behav, 32*(10), 2200-2210. doi:10.1016/j.addbeh.2007.02.011

Wimalawansa, S. J. (2014). Stigma of obesity: A major barrier to overcome(). *Journal of Clinical & Translational Endocrinology, 1*(3), 73-76. doi:10.1016/j.jcte.2014.06.001

Wu, Q., Wang, H., Fan, Y. Y., Zhang, J. M., Liu, X. Y., Fang, X. Y., Qi, Y. (2018). Ketogenic diet effects on 52 children with pharmacoresistant epileptic encephalopathy: A clinical prospective study. *Brain Behav, 8*(5), e00973. doi:10.1002/brb3.973

Yancy, W. S., Jr., Westman, E. C., McDuffie, J. R., Grambow, S. C., Jeffreys, A. S., Bolton, J., Oddone, E. Z. (2010). A randomized trial of a low-carbohydrate diet vs orlistat plus a low-fat diet for weight loss. *Arch Intern Med, 170*(2), 136-145. doi:10.1001/archinternmed.2009.492

Zhang, Y., Xu, J., Zhang, K., Yang, W., & Li, B. (2018). The Anticonvulsant Effects of Ketogenic Diet on Epileptic Seizures and Potential Mechanisms. *Curr Neuropharmacol, 16*(1), 66-70. doi:10.2174/1570159X15666170517153509

Zimmerman, G. L., Olsen, C. G., & Bosworth, M. F. (2000). A 'stages of change' approach to helping patients change behavior. *Am Fam Physician, 61*(5), 1409-1416.

Zinczenko, D., & Perrine, S. (2016). *Zero Sugar Diet: The 14-Day Plan to Flatten Your Belly, Crush Cravings, and Help Keep You Lean for Life*. New York: Ballantine.